HIGH PRAISE FOR THE JOYFUL ATHLETE

"Your book is tremendous. It has powerfully influenced my own practice, and I am recommending it to all my coaches plus our students in our Level 2 Precision Nutrition certification as part of a 'bodymind' curriculum unit."

> – **Krista Scott-Dixon**, Founder of Stumptuous.com (the leading strength training site for women)

"George Beinhorn and I have independently concluded that success in training (and life) comes from listening to your body and mind and finding your own ever-changing path to self-actualization. Eloquent and expansive in his exposition, Beinhorn has written an exceptional book for fitness-minded individuals of every persuasion."

> — **Clarence Bass, twice Mr. America** in his height and age class; author of the bodybuilding classic *RIPPED* and nine other books on leanness, fitness, and health—most recently, *Take Charge: Fitness at the Edge of Science*

"Based on scientific research, the experiences of elite runners, traditional training methods, and stories of athletes' experiences, this book clearly establishes the precedence of an expansive heart in harvesting power and joy from exercise and from all that we do."

> — **Michael Holland**, former Stanford University Specialty Coach for flexibility, strength, speed, power, and nutrition

"Beyond being a wonderful book, this is a doorway to new ways of training that can help us find joy. It's entertaining and readable, and the author writes beautifully. There are lots of people who could benefit from this information, but they won't find it anywhere else. I really, really enjoyed *The Joyful Athlete*.

> — **John Smallen**, marathon PR 2:37, 50 miles sub-7:00

"Since reading *The Joyful Athlete*, my daily aerobic exercise has become more interesting and rewarding on levels that go far beyond the body. This book showed me undreamed-of ways to get my mind, body, and spirit exercising in harmony. I believe it will help many people, and it's extremely well-written and enjoyable to read."

> —**Asha Praver**, recreational swimmer, inspirational speaker, author, *Loved and Protected*

THE JOYFUL
ATHLETE

THE WISDOM OF THE HEART
IN EXERCISE AND SPORTS TRAINING

George Beinhorn

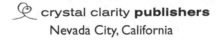
crystal clarity **publishers**
Nevada City, California

Crystal Clarity Publishers • Nevada City, CA 95959

ISBN 13: 978-1-56589-289-7
Epub ISBN 13: 978-1-56589-552-2

Cover Photograph © 2013 by George Beinhorn

Library of Congress
Cataloging-in-Publication Data *forthcoming*

 crystal clarity **publishers**
www.crystalclarity.com
800.424.1055 or 530.478.7600
clarity@crystalclarity.com

For SK

"Yes."

CONTENTS

PREFACE: SPIRITUAL MATTERS

In this book I refer, on rare occasions, to my relationship with a great spiritual teacher. At no point do I identify my spiritual path or my teacher's name. And that's deliberate. The principles of sports training are the same whether we follow Christ, Buddha, Zoroaster, Moses, Yogananda, Muhammed, or no one.

Expansive values of kindness, compassion, and love are prized in all spiritual traditions. They are universal. And it's impossible to talk about success in sports without mentioning these positive dimensions of the human heart. Research that I cite in chapter 5, "Science of the Heart," shows that feelings such as kindness and compassion are intimately related to sports performance. For example, expansive feelings make the heart beat in an efficient rhythm that allows us to exercise harder with less strain.

I believe this book will help followers of any path, or no path. In these pages, you'll discover how elite athletes, coaches, and scientists are confirming that positive thoughts and feelings and success go together.

1. THE SIMPLE JOY OF SPORTS

During a vacation in Hawaii last summer, I picked up a hitchhiker on Kauai's north shore. He was a fit-looking young man in his early twenties who spoke with a French accent. He told me he'd grown up in Tahiti but was living in France, and that he was a professional body-boarder. I asked if he rode big waves. He said, "Yeah, that's my thing—it takes lots of wave-energy to perform well."

He told me he'd grown tired of the endless travel his sport required, and that he was thinking of taking a break, because he was no longer happy being a professional athlete. His voice thickening with regret, he described how riding the waves as a child in Tahiti had been pure joy, and how competition had sapped that pristine happiness.

"Competing, you have to play tricks on your friends," he said. "You can't even talk to them the same way anymore."

I marveled—this young man had accomplished so much, and already he was career-weary. And some moxie, too, to drop off a two-story wall of water while performing tricks along the way. His voice was firm with the resolution that had made his accomplishments possible.

We talked in a general way about sports, and I mentioned that I'd worked at *Runner's World* in the early 1970s. I told him about a conversation I'd had with Joe Henderson, the magazine's founding editor, while we ran ten miles together during a recent marathon.

Joe talked about the changes in running over the last four decades. In the seventies, when the Americans were competitive at the highest level, many were friends who trained together and shared their methods, even as the world-dominating Kenyans do today. Joe said that with big money riding on every race, the Americans no longer feel comfortable hanging out and sharing their secrets.

I told the body boarder that I'd spent much of my vacation snorkeling at Tunnels Lagoon. His voice rose with excitement as he described the "amazing numbers of seashells" I would find if I swam straight out from the singer Charo's house to a gap in the reef where the currents drop piles of debris. "You'll find many wonderful things!" he said, his pleasure in sharing contrasting with the weary tones in which he'd described his career impasse.

I told him how, while I was at *Runner's World*, I would often photograph indoor track meets that would start with races for elementary school kids, and how the crowd would go wild, screaming and whistling as the tiny kids flailed around the track. I told him how it had struck me that the applause for the professionals was always more subdued.

The body boarder appeared to resent my saying this, as if I'd cast a slur on his sport. "I *like* competition," he said sullenly, as he stepped out of the car.

I regretted that I hadn't been able to explain my meaning more clearly. Putting down his sport was the last thing on my mind. I'd simply wanted to share a feeling that audiences respond more enthusiastically to a certain naïve joy in sports, than to events tinged with too much adult hype and seriousness.

Reflecting on our conversation, I wondered if the young

body-boarder's simple happiness riding the waves as a boy hadn't helped him rise to the top of his sport. If he could recover some of that unselfconscious joy, perhaps he could forget about his opponents and perform better than ever. It might take courage, because he'd have to become inwardly engrossed in pure play again, and less focused on external rewards. Going his own way, he might find himself further distanced from his competitors. But his purity would surely win their respect in the end, and his joy might even inspire them.

An idealistic scenario? A Pollyanna-ish ending for a Hollywood film script? Possibly.

When Michael Jordan joined the Chicago Bulls, he insisted on a clause in his contract that spelled out his freedom to play basketball whenever and wherever he liked, including joining in neighborhood pickup games. And when a reporter asked then-Bulls coach Phil Jackson to characterize Jordan's co-star Scottie Pippen in a single phrase, Jackson thought for a moment and replied: "The joy of basketball."

In sports nowadays, joy can be hard to find. Turning on the TV, the odds are good that we'll be treated to the sight of professional athletes whining, brawling, and preening. Numbed by the parade of boorishness, we gloss over behaviors that would have brought a blush to the cheeks of the great philosopher-coaches: people like Vince Lombardi, Jim Counsilman, John Wooden, Bill Walsh, Dean Smith, and George Halas.

As fans, we may have to take what's dished out to us. But as participants, we can craft our own experiences. Like Jordan and Pippen, we can make a conscious decision to turn sports, at our level, into a quest for expansion—an artistic performance, a daily celebration, a spiritual search for joy.

How can we experience pure joy in sports? We can learn a lot from great athletes who've shown exceptional qualities as people.

Granted this is personal, but I'm inspired when I see Ann Trason, the greatest female ultramarathon runner of all time, handing out cups of Gatorade at an obscure trail race in the hills north of San Francisco, motivated by the simple pleasure of helping old geezers like me.

I'm inspired by Mark Plaatjes, winner of the 1993 World Championships marathon. During the New York City marathon the following year, Plaatjes was running with the lead pack when an injury forced him to drop out. Instead of retreating to his hotel room to sulk, he hobbled to the nearest aid station, where he volunteered his skills as a physical therapist to massage the slower runners.

Aside from their amazing physical gifts, what are some of the traits that inspire us in great athletes? Gymnast Kerri Strug's courageous performance at the 1996 Olympics comes to mind. With an injured ankle, Strug performed a vault that ensured a gold medal for her team. Surely, an inspiring quality in athletes is a heart that's big enough to include others in its sympathy.

Loving, expansive feelings aren't exclusive to great athletes, of course, but can an athlete be considered truly great without them?

Consider Ty Cobb. I first learned of the professional baseball Hall of Famer's career when I was seven or eight years old. I happened to mention his amazing lifetime batting average to my father, and to my surprise, Dad fell silent. I knew from this that there was something vaguely wrong about Cobb, but it would be 45 years before I learned of his darker side, when I watched Ken Burns's *Baseball* documentary on PBS.

It dawned on me then that my father had been unwilling to discuss Cobb's faults, however reprehensible, and that it was a mark of Dad's goodness that he'd been reluctant to do so.

But, hey, let's be realistic. Sure, everyone loves a jock with a heart of gold, but can athletes truly afford to harbor big, floppy feelings? Can an NFL linebacker afford to love his competitors? If he treats them with kindness, won't they cheerfully murder him on the spot? *(Certainly.)* On third and goal, there's not much room for politeness: *"Yo—after you!" "No, no—after you!"* Whether winning requires beating the crap out of someone may depend on the sport. But there's solid scientific evidence that expansive attitudes contribute to athletic success, and not merely by distracting us from energy-draining negativity.

A review of 101 studies of several thousand men and women revealed that negative emotions can have severe health consequences:

People who experienced chronic anxiety, long periods of sadness and pessimism, unremitting tension or incessant hostility, relentless cynicism or suspiciousness, were found to have *double* the risk of disease—including asthma, arthritis, headaches, peptic ulcers, and heart disease (each representative of major, broad categories of disease).[1]

As 1972 Olympic marathon gold medalist Frank Shorter put it, "The marathon is too hard a race to waste energy hating your competitors." The same could be said of any difficult sport—life included.

At a recent business meeting, I was introduced to a former

---

1. Daniel Goleman, *Emotional Intelligence* (New York: Bantam Books, 1997), 168–69. The study mentioned is: Howard Friedman and Stephanie Boothby-Kewley, "The Disease-Prone Personality: A Meta-Analytic View," *American Psychologist* 42 (1987).

college football player for whom the consequences of negative attitudes had taken a particularly brutal turn. He'd been an All-American linebacker at a nationally ranked NCAA Division I school. In his playing days, he'd weighed 245 pounds, and he'd had a 20-inch neck. When I met him, he looked like a tennis player—slim, athletic, well-proportioned, but nothing like his former hulking self.

He told me about a game he'd played, where a 300-pound offensive tackle had given him a difficult time. Frustrated and angry, he chose his moment and deliberately hit his nemesis in the knees, disabling him and sending him off the field. "He didn't give me any more trouble," he said. "I saw him several years later when I transferred to his school. He was hobbling across the campus using a cane."

He then told me how, after graduation, he'd been in a terrible car accident that left him completely paralyzed. The doctors put him in a metal frame with buttons he could push to move around. His body wasted away. When I met him, he'd spent years painstakingly rebuilding his fitness to the point where he could walk and ride a bicycle.

We didn't discuss the subtle karmic payback mechanism that may have been involved. But it was obvious from the way he described his experiences that he believed he'd incurred a serious debt in ending the lineman's career, and that the bill had come due with a vengeance. The American nineteenth-century philosopher Ralph Waldo Emerson was probably right when he described a "law of compensation" that rewards us according to our deeds.

In his fine book, *Running with the Legends*, journalist Michael Sandrock compares the ever-cheerful Frank Shorter, whose phenomenal career spanned 10 years of racing at the highest level, with Australian Derek Clayton, the former marathon world record holder (2:08:33), whose career was plagued by injuries, thanks to his ruthless approach to training.

Just as with [British Olympic marathoner Ron] Hill, there is something in Shorter's makeup that set him apart from Clayton. A story that gives an idea of Clayton's personality is one he tells when speaking at prerace clinics. Clayton relates how during a race, he missed his drink at an aid station. A Japanese competitor running alongside graciously offered Clayton his own bottle. After taking some of the drink, Clayton began to hand it back to the Japanese runner. Suddenly, he changed his mind. Instead of giving it back to the Japanese runner, Clayton turned and threw the bottle off to the side of the road. Clayton was proud of that, and of the fact that he trained so hard that he would sometimes be "pissing blood."

Sandrock observes, "Lots of runners train hard, but only the select few are able to put it together when it counts." Meaning, presumably, that a ruthless attitude doesn't always win the race. At the 1972 Olympics where Shorter won gold, Clayton finished a disappointed thirteenth.

US Olympian Kenny Moore relates a telling story about Shorter:

Having been drafted and temporarily assigned to the Army track team, I'd finished third behind Jack Bacheler and Juan Martinez in the six-mile and qualified for the US team going to Europe. Afterward, I'd gone to talk to the feather-footed guy in a Yale uniform whom I'd sat on all the way and outkicked with a violent, 26-second last 200. "Sorry about that," I said. "If I didn't make the team, it was infantry training and Nam for me."

"Jesus Christ!" said Frank Shorter, "Why didn't you

say something? We could have worked it out. You didn't have to kill yourself like that." That was the beginning of a beautiful friendship.[2]

Our everyday experiences tell us that contractive feelings sap our energy. Shorter was right: life is too hard to waste precious resources hating others. Moreover, the notion that expansive feelings such as love and kindness promote health and improve performance is no longer an airy sentiment. It's been verified by the discovery of electrical and chemical pathways by which the effects of our positive and negative thoughts and feelings are carried to the most distant parts of our bodies, including the immune system, which is vitally involved in sports training and recovery.

Bruce Ogilvy, PhD, a pioneering sports psychologist, once studied the factors that had prevented a group of world-class badminton players from rising to the top of their sport. Ogilvy found that the second-tier athletes tended to beat themselves up mentally for their mistakes, while the champions simply noted their errors and moved on, wasting no energy on self-recrimination. The top players inwardly reviewed their flubs and quickly turned to the next task. Negative self-thoughts sap our energy. They are self-defeating.

Is it surprising, then, that so many great players, including Michael Jordan, have remained positive and expansive, relishing the game until the end of their careers? In his wonderful biography, *Playing for Keeps—Michael Jordan & the World He Made*, David Halberstam ties Jordan's phenomenal success to his happy spirit:

Jordan seemed almost innately joyous. His pleasure seemed to come from playing basketball, and he generated

2. Kenny Moore, *Bowerman and the Men of Oregon: The Story of Oregon's Legendary Coach and Nike's Cofounder* (Emmaus, PA: Rodale Press, 2005), 236.

the most natural kind of self-confidence. . . .

He was going to be a great player, Loughery [Jordan's college roommate] thought, not just because of the talent and the uncommon physical assets but because he loved the game. That love could not be coached or faked, and it was something he always had. He was joyous about practices, joyous about games, as if he could not wait for either. Not many players had that kind of love. All too many modern players, Loughery believed, loved the money instead of the game. But Jordan's love of what he did was real, and it was a huge advantage.

In Jordan's words:

People talk about my work ethic as a player, but they don't understand. What appeared to be hard work to others was simply playing for me. We were playing a game. Why not play as hard as you can? There's no pressure in taking that approach.[3]

A cornerstone of the world's spiritual teachings holds that each time we make our awareness a little bit larger, our soul—the internal conduit for God's infinite bliss—rewards us with a corresponding little extra shot of joy. Spiritual teachings tell us that cultivating expansive, positive thoughts and feelings promotes health and well-being, while negative thoughts and emotions poison the body and make it vulnerable to disease.

If joyful, expansive attitudes can spread good vibrations throughout our bodies, surely they won't stand in the way of sports performance, and they may, in fact, give us a powerful advantage. In every area of our lives, positive, life-affirming attitudes are a key to success: in relationships, business, child-raising, and exercise. Even if our goal is just to lose ten pounds, our joy in the achievement will be amplified if we

3. Mark Vancil, ed., *Driven From Within*, (New York: Atria Books, 2005), 18.

can devise ways to shed the pounds "expansively"—perhaps to the end of having more energy for our family and friends.

It isn't hard to understand how expansion works. Consider the experience of people who start an exercise program. After the first few uncomfortable weeks, they find that they can climb stairs, take out the garbage, and play with the kids with greater zest and freedom. As fresh energy spreads throughout their being, they find themselves feeling happier, more mentally alert and in tune with the life around them. Where they were formerly dragged down and confined by the torporous mass of their own flesh, they now have visions of surfing on waves of energy. Their awareness—the range and force of their bodies, hearts, and minds—has expanded.

Spiritual teachings tell us that these welcome increases of happiness are mere hints of an even greater expansion of joy that awaits us, as we extend our awareness sufficiently to loosen the ego's grip and open our hearts to God's boundless love and bliss.

I'm certainly not going to claim that every successful athlete is a quivering mass of joy. I read a newspaper story recently about a 270-pound college football player who, enraged because his fast-food order hadn't included *chalupas*, tried to attack the attendant and became stuck in the service window, from which he had to be extricated by the police.

To expect every successful athlete to be a model of compassion and humility would be—well, stupid. Basketball player Charles Barkley nailed it, in the famous Nike commercial where he intones: *"I am not your role model."*

Still, there are excellent grounds for believing that athletes who *are* expansive get more from their sport, at least in the dimensions of their being where they're expansive. (Whether they perform better is up to science to decide.) It may not take loving feelings to win the Super Bowl, but if you can get through the battle with some part of your essential humanity intact, who's to doubt that it will add a positive dimension to the experience.

Consider the great philosopher-coaches mentioned earlier. Take Jim Counsilman, the swimming coach who built a dynasty of NCAA-champion teams at the University of Indiana. Counsilman worked tirelessly to combat selfishness and narrow-heartedness among his swimmers. He devoted a great deal of ingenuity to making their workouts fun, because he believed that a relaxed atmosphere, colored with positive, expansive feelings enhances athletic performance.

Or take John Wooden, the legendary UCLA basketball coach whose teams dominated the NCAA in the 1960s and '70s, winning 10 national championships. The UCLA players were required to study Wooden's famous "Pyramid of Success," which included such expansive values as "cooperation," "enthusiasm," "loyalty," "friendship," and "team spirit." Wooden's autobiography, *My Personal Best: Life Lessons from an All-American Journey*, published in 2004 when he was 94, is one of the most inspiring sports books of all time. There's a wonderful video, *Values, Victory and Peace of Mind*, in which the "Wizard of Westwood," still clear-eyed at 90, presents the Pyramid, with respectful appearances from former UCLA players Bill Walton and Kareem Abdul-Jabbar, and NBA coach Phil Jackson.

Even Vince Lombardi, the notoriously tough-minded coach who led the Green Bay Packers to victory in the first Super Bowl, practiced expansive values when it counted. Lombardi wasn't hard on his players only to get the best out of them on the field. Bart Starr, the Packers' Hall of Fame quarterback, recalls:

He never treated football as an end result, but rather a means to an end. He was concerned with the full, total life. . . . . Tough, demanding, abrasive, he was also compassionate and understanding. For though he recognized that absolute perfection is never attainable, he believed the quest for it can be one of the most challenging races an individual can run.

Jerry Kramer, the Packers' All-Pro guard, put it more bluntly: "I had hated him at times during training camp and I had hated him at times during the season, but I knew how much he had done for us, and I knew how much he cared about us. He is a beautiful man."

Joe Ehrmann is a former Baltimore Colts All-Pro defensive tackle. Ehrman now coaches high school football at the Gilman School in Baltimore. He believes young athletes today are encouraged to grow up believing in three wrong values: athletic ability, sexual conquest, and economic success. He calls these "false masculinity."

"Masculinity, first and foremost, ought to be defined in terms of relationships," Joe said. "It ought to be taught in terms of the capacity to *love* and to *be* loved. . . . And I think the second criterion—the only other criterion for masculinity—is that all of us ought to have some kind of cause, some kind of purpose in our lives that's bigger than our own individual hopes, dreams, wants, and desires."[4]

Ehrmann teaches his players a code of conduct that's starkly at variance with the values most young athletes absorb. It includes accepting responsibility, leading courageously, and "enacting justice on behalf of others." Ehrmann's "Building Men for Others" program is based on empathy: "Not feeling

---

4. Jeffrey Marx, *Season of Life: A Football Star, A Boy, A Journey to Manhood* (Simon & Schuster, 2003).

for someone, but *with* someone."

Biff Poggi, head football coach at Gilman, read a newspaper article that quoted the coach at another school: "You have to push them [high school football players] to the brink and either they are going to break or they are going to stand up and be a man."

Poggi took the article to a team meeting, where he read it aloud to the players and chortled:

"We ought to get a lifetime contract to play against this guy. We'd beat them every time we'd play, because he has no idea what he's talking about. You understand? Fifty boys together, fifty boys that love each other and that are well affirmed and well loved by their coaches, will smack those guys anytime, in *anything*. Being a father. Being a son. Being a football player. Being a doctor. Being an astronaut. Being a human being. Being anything.

"That's *not* how you become a man. Do you understand me? Because that means to be a man, you gotta somehow be some big, strong, physical person. And that's got nothing to do with it. Trust me."[5]

When *Season of Life* was written, Gilman had been state champion two seasons in a row, winning all their games and ranking among the nation's top ten high school teams.

Dean Ottati is a friend and the author of an entertaining and insightful book, *The Runner and the Path*. A high school football team in Dean's hometown of Concord, California, the De La Salle Spartans, set the record for the longest unbeaten streak in high school history, winning 151 straight games in 13 years (1991–2004), while holding the number-one national ranking for much of that time.

Dean was getting his hair cut one day and talking about

---

5. Ibid.

the team with the barber. Dean said, "There's no way they don't recruit players from other schools."

A woman sitting in the shop overheard Dean's remark. She said, "Let me tell you something. My son played for De La Salle, and I would be willing to *die* for Coach Lad [De La Salle head football coach Bob Ladouceur]. I would do anything for that man, for what he did for my son."

Like Joe Ehrmann, Coach Ladouceur teaches values of brotherhood, sportsmanship, and integrity. The fact is, De La Salle doesn't have to recruit, because parents are dying to get their sons into the school, not only for football but for the values they'll absorb. The Spartans are the subject of an inspiring book, *When the Game Stands Tall: The Story of the De La Salle Spartans and Football's Longest Winning Streak*, by Neil Hayes.

———————— o ————————

My best performances as a runner are not impressive. Almost 40 years ago, at age 32, I ran a 5K in 18 minutes, a mediocre time, and it like to killed me. I've never been able to run 400 meters faster than 73 seconds. At age 53, after training hard for seven months, I eked out a 10-mile race in 70 minutes, thereby earning no bragging rights. In my mid-twenties, I spent three years paralyzed from the chest down (a benign tumor was compressing my spinal cord), and although I recovered, my legs still aren't hooked up right. My left leg has lingering spasticity and my right leg is mildly paralyzed. Meet Spaz and Gumby. The surgeries left me with a near-constant feeling as if my brain and heart are cross-wired and short-circuited. I've got the body of a great African runner, all right: the biomechanics of a rhino and the VO_2Max of a tree sloth. Yet I find that I can experience joy fairly reliably when I run, by cultivating an expansive attitude.

In fact, it's a feature of the law of expansion that you don't have to be fast, young, or gifted to make it work. You don't even have to be fit, because you can taste the joys of expanded awareness by "nudging your edges" in any dimension of your being: body, heart, will, mind, soul. You've met people like that—men and women who were overweight and unhealthy, but who were joyful in areas of their lives where they expressed expansive qualities of kindness, courage, and love.

Several weeks ago, I had an unusual experience while running at Rancho San Antonio, a beautiful park in the foothills of the San Francisco Peninsula.

For the last seven years I'd run ultramarathons. I was feeling the need for a change, but I was uncertain what to do. As I ran, I prayed, saying, "What's next? What should I do now?"

I was surprised to hear the clear intuitive voice of my spiritual teacher. It said, with powerful emphasis, almost shouting: *"Retire!!!"*

The message struck a chord. The six- and seven-hour training runs required by the ultramarathon sport were taking a toll on my work and relationships. At the same time, it was discouraging. I'd invested so many years, run thousands of miles—and for what? *"Retire!"* sounded ominously like quitting. But what could I look *forward* to?

A week later, I was thinking about this again during a 10-mile run in the hills behind Stanford University. I was feeling a little down—I certainly didn't want to quit. If that's what "retire" meant, it wasn't a pill I could happily swallow.

Emerging from the hills onto a nearby street, I felt a freshness enter my legs and I picked up the pace, feeling surprisingly joyful. Soon I was cruising at a fast clip, light and smooth, my spirits rising.

Turning my attention inward, I asked what it meant, and once again I heard the intuitive voice. This time it said, *"Do you think you'd be feeling this way, if I meant that you should retire completely from running?"*

Several miles later, near the end of the run, I was warming down, jogging slowly and feeling a bit sandbagged. I passed a grassy field where three Stanford soccer players, a woman and two men, were practicing a ball-control drill. The players were rimmed in golden light by the late-afternoon sun and backlit against the green grass. For some reason the scene captured my attention, and I slowed to watch.

A player ran toward an orange plastic pylon, then cut back sharply while a second player tossed him the ball; the first player then kicked the ball into the arms of the third player. They repeated the drill over and over, with relentless skill and fully absorbed attention, and for reasons I can't begin to explain, my heart was flooded with joy. The scene seemed to embody the Zen concept of "suchness"—it was a thing complete in itself, a small miracle of beauty and economy, and I nearly wept with happiness. My fatigue vanished, and I sailed through a nearby eucalyptus grove on legs as light as air.

A moment of simple magic had released an energy and joy that washed away my fatigue away. What if I could run like that again and again? Could I banish fatigue by expanding my heart to the point of self-forgetfulness? What lessons would I have to learn to be able to repeat the experience at will?

Casting my mind back over my four decades as a runner, I realized that I had experienced a similar joy on many occasions—as an inner warmth of heart, or a fusion of energy and silence. And always those moments had come when I succeeded in opening doors through which my awareness could escape the narrow confines of the little ego and emerge into a wider reality.

My life as a runner had taught me a simple lesson: expansion equals joy. I no longer felt discouraged about letting go of ultramarathoning.

The spiritual teachings of the world tell us that life offers endless opportunities for expansion into a greater happiness. As one teacher put it, "You go on until you achieve endlessness." I realized there was much to look forward to.

2. INTRODUCTION: HEART TALK

I've always felt that the best training is the kind that delivers rewards both inwardly and outwardly—where our fitness increases, and our exercise becomes increasingly enjoyable.

What's the best training to achieve those results? I spent several decades searching for the answer. And I gradually came to understand that the "method" is both simple and complex.

Simple, because really, it's just asking a fairly straightforward question: "What's the best way to train?"

In my experience, when our training is in harmony with our body's needs, the "joy of sports" follows naturally.

But training well is also complex, because it demands that we answer five tough questions:

1. *Body.* How can I fine-tune my training in harmony with my body's ever-changing needs?

2. *Heart.* How can I find the joy of expansive feelings when I train?

3. *Will.* How can I train with strong will, without getting injured or over-trained?

4. *Mind.* How can I focus and quiet my mind, so I can enter the enjoyable sports "zone"?

5. *Soul.* How can I commune with the wisdom and joy of a higher intelligence when I exercise?

At this point, I wouldn't be surprised if you're feeling suspicious. Perhaps you suspect that the "formula" will prove to be extremely complex, that it will take 300 pages to explain, and that there will be a copout in the final pages. Yet, as I promised above, the answer to those five challenging questions turns out to be surprisingly simple. Let me explain.

Where do athletes generally turn when they have questions about their training? I suspect most of us consult three sources:

Science. We read articles and books by respected sports scientists, and we do as they recommend.

Trial and error. We thumb through the pages of our training diary, and we repeat what worked in the past.

The experiences of others. We read what successful athletes and coaches have done, and we imitate them.

There's a lot to be said for each approach. But notice that just one—trial and error—addresses the unique needs of the individual athlete. Even so, the most meticulous training diary can only tell us what worked when conditions were nearly (they're never exactly) the same as they are today.

Let's look more closely at the first approach—science— since it's probably the one athletes trust the most.

There are thousands of books and articles on training, based on sports science. Yet I've always felt that there's an important element that they tend to leave out.

Articles for runners, for example, tell us over and over how to improve our 10K and marathon times, based on the latest scientific research.[6] But they don't tell us much about how to fine-tune our training "on the fly," from moment to moment, during each and every run. Yet, as every newcomer

---

6. In this book I refer to running, since it's the sport I'm most familiar with. However, I believe the *principles* of expansive athletics apply to all sports.

soon discovers, rigidly following inflexible training schedules is a recipe for disaster, because each body is unique, and the body's needs change continually.

Science looks at the *outside* of sports. It studies the body as a working machine. Science describes an imaginary "average" body, based on poking and prodding hundreds of bodies. But when we look under the hood at the *individual* body, the picture becomes vastly more complex.

The body that *we* must train with isn't a scientifically averaged body; it's a specific organism that reacts in unique ways to the countless factors that may affect it on a given day: our sleep patterns and diet, the weather, yesterday's training, our stress level at work and home, and so on. Not to mention the factors we're born with and can't change: our VO_2Max, biodynamics, etc.

When it comes to planning our training, clearly it's the individual body that counts. Yet the sports scientists hardly ever tell us how to "listen to our bodies." Certainly, they advise us to take our morning pulse and monitor other physical markers of overtraining. But they don't tell us how to listen to our bodies moment by moment, so that we can avoid overtraining in the first place.

Don't get me wrong, I'm not "against" science. Science has given us wonderful insights about how our bodies work. But it hasn't done a very good job of telling us how to *individualize* our training.

In *Lore of Running* (4th ed.), Timothy Noakes, MD, one of the world's most respected sports scientists, makes a startling admission:

Surprisingly few studies of the effects of different training regimes on athletic performance have been quantified in scientifically designed trials. In part, this is because few exercise scientists have considered this to be important, choosing rather to study how the body adapts to training at the cellular and molecular level. Perhaps they believe that neither the Nobel Prize in Physiology or Medicine nor its sporting equivalent, the International Olympic Committee Science Prize, will be won by the exercise scientist who first discovers the most ideal athletic training program.

Just hours ago, I read an article in the *New York Times* about research that discredits the lactic-acid theory of fatigue, which for 80 years was considered an unassailable pillar of sports science. It seems that lactic acid doesn't "cause fatigue" after all, as we were led to believe. In fact, lactic acid is an important fuel for the working muscles.

From the *Times* article:

"It's one of the classic mistakes in the history of science," Dr. Brooks said. [George A. Brooks, professor of integrative biology at the University of California, Berkeley] . . . .

Yet, Dr. Brooks said, even though coaches often believed in the myth of the lactic acid threshold, they ended up training athletes in the best way possible to increase their mitochondria. "Coaches have understood things the scientists didn't," he said.

Through trial and error, coaches learned that athletic performance improved when athletes worked on endurance, running longer and longer distances, for example.

That, it turns out, increased the mass of their muscle mitochondria, letting them burn more lactic acid and allowing the muscles to work harder and longer.[7]

---

7. Gina Kolata, "Lactic Acid Is Not Muscles' Foe, It's Fuel," *New*

If science can't tell us everything we need to know about training, we're left with little choice but to "train empirically"—that is, conduct our own experiments and figure out what works best for our own unique, individual body. And that may not be a bad thing.

In a *Runner's World Daily* interview, David L. Costill, an internationally renowned sports physiologist, put it like this: "The best computer in the world is in your head. The experience of training, of running a race. You learn what the thresholds are."[8]

Tom Osler, a legendary ultramarathoner and author of a classic book on training, wrote:

Science is wonderful (as a mathematician, I am one of her servants myself), but she has her limitations. Frankly, I believe running is far too complicated for successful technical analysis at this time. It is the runners themselves, through their direct empirical findings, who will point the way for the professional physiologist and rarely, very rarely, that the physiologist will provide practical knowledge of use to the competing athlete. In the words of the great mathematician and engineer Oliver Heaviside, "One does not need to understand the physiology of digestion in order to enjoy a good meal."[9]

In fact, all of the most successful training systems have been derived empirically. Arthur Lydiard, the legendary

York Times, May 16, 2006. Downloaded from http://www.nytimes.com/2006/05/16/health/nutrition/ 16run.html?ex=1148011200&en=e ef2896c5c908265&ei=5070 on May 17, 2006.

8. Downloaded from http://runnersworld.com/article/0,712 ,s6-243-292—10704-0,00.html on October 26, 2006.

9. Tom Osler, *Serious Runner's Handbook* (Mountain View, CA: World Publications, 1978), 11–12.

coach whose methods were adopted by successive waves of Olympic champions from New Zealand, Australia, Japan, Finland, Mexico, Africa, and the US, evolved his ideas by first testing them on himself.

When Lydiard wanted to know the best weekly training mileage for a talented distance runner, for example, he ran 80 to 300 miles a week and painstakingly tracked the results. Based on countless experiments conducted in the laboratory of his own body, Lydiard evolved the systems of "periodization" and "peaking" that would dominate the training of world-class runners for two decades, and that are enjoying a revival today.

In a talk that Lydiard gave in Japan shortly before his death in January 2005, he emphasized the need to adapt our training to our own, individual requirements, and to avoid relying too heavily on the blanket advice of others:

> One of the reasons why Americans don't produce very many good middle distance and distance runners, with millions of people there running, is simply because of this factor: coaches determining with hypothetical figures exactly what athletes should do in anaerobic training. Well, as a coach, you may be able to determine pretty closely what your athlete can do. You may be right in saying he can do fifteen 400 meters in 65 seconds with such-and-such interval. But the main thing is to explain to the athlete not only how and what to do, but why he is doing it. What physiological reactions he is to bring about with the training. And when he finishes, when he hits the wall, he's had enough. And he should determine when to stop, not the coach. *The key to training is to train to your individual reactions to the training.* [Italics mine.]

Speaking in Boulder, Colorado on December 2, 2004,

Lydiard said: "You need to find your own limits. Everyone wants to know how much, how fast. They want it on a piece of paper. *Your conditions change every day.*" [Italics mine.]

We really have no choice but to make training a personal experiment—monitoring our body's reactions and adjusting our training accordingly. But the immediate question then becomes: "How will my body tell me what it can handle? And how can I 'hear' what it says?"

Everything is limited by the body. You can never advance your training faster than your body's ability to recover. And some bodies take longer to recover than others. You can only train as hard as *your own individual* body can manage. It cannot be emphasized strongly enough: every body is unique. Thus, it's extremely important to find a way to "listen to the body"—to know, with certainty, what your unique body's needs are, day by day, so that you can train accordingly.

What instrument can tell us, clearly and unmistakably, the kind of training that will keep the body healthy and nudge it to improve?

It's easy to know *after* a run if you've done too much or too little. That's why we keep a training diary: to learn, over the weeks, months, and years, how our bodies generally react to different kinds of training. The diary can help us make better decisions, based on experience and common sense. But what if there were also a way to know *while* we're running, if what we're doing is exactly right?

I'm not recommending that you throw your diary away, or abandon your common sense and reason. But one of the best tools I've found for knowing what will improve my fitness and the inner quality of my runs is intuition—the calm, impartial feelings of the heart.

Many years ago, I began to notice that the subtle feelings

of my heart were trying to tell me the kind of training my body "wanted" or could handle on a given day. At first, I brushed those messages aside impatiently, because they often seemed to be telling me things I didn't want to hear—like *Slow down!*—or *Pack it in!*—or *Go home!* Also, because I thought it was kind of airy-fairy to be running around "listening to my heart." But when I began to take those signals seriously, I began having deeply enjoyable runs more often, and I was able to make better decisions about my training.

In time, I realized that paying attention to the heart wasn't "airy-fairy" at all—that logic and feeling complement each other; that they are both indispensable tools.

A common prejudice in our reason-dominant culture says that we can follow *either* reason *or* feeling, but not both. Partly, of course, it's true—in fact, *emotional* feeling can be very misleading. Yet a landmark study that I'll cite in chapter 6 ("Focus on Feeling") found that people whose brains were damaged by physical trauma, impairing their ability to feel, had a terrible time making decisions, even though their reasoning powers were intact.

The "either/or" dogma—*either* feeling *or* reason—is simply wrong. For starters, it doesn't take into account that there are different *kinds* of feeling. The type of intuitive feeling I'm talking about, which can help us make good decisions, isn't personal or wildly emotional; it's calm, *impersonal* feeling. It's the kind of feeling you experience when you face an important decision, and you say: "Let me set aside my emotions and prejudices and get inwardly calm and feel what's *right.*"

There's nothing terribly mystical or spooky about intuition—although it definitely extends into spiritual realms. We use intuition all the time in our daily lives, even if we don't call it by that name.

Imagine that you're trying to decide which of two equally qualified job candidates to hire. One candidate gives you a good feeling, and the other makes you nervous, though you can't put your finger on exactly why.

Or imagine that your spouse suggests that you travel to her parents' for Thanksgiving. You agree, but on some deep level of your awareness, you know you won't be going. Sure enough, your youngest child falls ill and the trip is canceled.

You respond to an ad for a used computer. You drive to the seller's home, where everything seems fine. But you have an uneasy feeling—a whisper of intuition that seems to be telling you "Don't do it." With regret, you leave without buying. The next day, you find a more capable PC for less money.

Here's an experiment in intuition that you can try whenever you face a critical decision:

Stop what you're doing. "Call time out." Go to a quiet place where you feel relaxed and undistracted—perhaps a nearby park. Find a place where you feel comfortable and calm, where you can be yourself.

Sit for a while and relax. Be grateful for the break in your day. Savor it, and when you're feeling calm, turn your attention to the decision before you, and review the alternatives. As you contemplate each option, check the feeling in your heart. Try to find a calm, impartial level of feeling that isn't affected by personal prejudices and desires. Chances are, one choice will generate a more positive, upbeat feeling than the others.

That's the first step. The next is to act on the feeling—but tentatively. Take a step forward and check the feeling again. Be aware that with each step the "landscape" will change, with fresh decisions to be made. If your heart is calm, moving forward in one direction will feel subtly "right," while the other choices will evoke a subtle sense of disharmony or "wrongness."

Warning: Don't try this with really big decisions!—at least not until you've had plenty of practice. Decisions about relationships, cars, and computers are seldom easy to contemplate with a calm heart.

In fact, the most difficult part of using intuition is persuading the heart to be calm and impartial.

There are many ways to improve your ability to hear the intuitive messages your body is sending. For example, research I'll describe in chapter 6 shows that anything you can do to generate harmonious, happy feelings in your heart will improve ability to focus your mind, be calmly impartial, and know what's right.

Throughout this book, I'll suggest ways to generate those positive, expansive feelings while you run. And I'll describe some of my own struggles to find that detached, intuitive place in my heart.

If you take just one message from this book, I hope it will be this: when you're looking for the intuitive, happy part of your heart, don't try to get there with your *mind*. Trying to *think* your way to a state of intuitive feeling doesn't work. Instead, go straight to the heart.

The quickest way to find the intuitive heart is by using "heart-means." Do whatever makes you *feel* happy, calm and expansive, whether it's singing, remembering a happy experience, thinking of a friend, sending silent blessings to loved ones, or opening your heart to the rhythms of running, or to nature, or Spirit.

If your thoughts are scattered or unhappy at the start of a run, don't waste time *thinking and worrying* about it, generating endless words. Instead, run your way into a happier "place." (For more suggestions, see chapter 4, "The

Harmony Zone.") When we're deeply *interested* in what we're doing, the mind naturally and effortlessly finds a focus. Trying to *force* the mind to concentrate is nearly always a waste of time. The deepest concentration comes when we're relaxed and engaged.

Let your thoughts wander and grouse, if they must. Just run. Let the rhythm of running, the movement of your footfall and breathing, soothe your mind and heart until you feel more centered and cheerful. As you cultivate good feelings, the mind will follow.

In fact, it's a time-tested rule: "The mind tends to follow whatever feeling is uppermost in the heart." When we feel something strongly, the mind tends to trot along and support that feeling. If you have a hankering for ice cream, for example, you'll find your mind obediently supplying all the logical reasons why ice cream would be a really good thing for you to have *right now*. When you feel blue, your mind lists all the ways life is cruel and unfair, and why the world owes you more than it's giving. Isn't it so?

In this book, I'll suggest ways you can *use* your mind to stimulate positive feelings that will help you relax, focus, and hear your body's intuitive whispers. In all of these practices, it's good to be "intense, but not tense." *Relax!* It's not just important; it's essential.

Many years ago, when I began to be aware that my body was trying to talk to me through my heart, I discovered that there was a running pace at which those messages were easiest to hear. I call that pace the "harmony zone." I'll say more about it in chapter 4. For now, here's a preview.

The harmony zone is a subjective experience—it's an actual "happy feeling" in the area of the heart. It's a subtle, enjoyable feeling of "rightness" that tells me I'm doing exactly the right thing, the thing that's healthiest for my body, and that will improve my fitness most efficiently. Those happy feelings show up when I run at the pace my body "wants" on the day—the harmony zone pace. If I ignore the signals and run too hard or too far, the good feelings fade, replaced by a subtle disharmony.

Listening to my body's wisdom, speaking through the "voice" of the intuitive heart, I find I can apply scientific training methods more wisely, with better awareness of my body's unique needs.

Jeff Galloway, a U.S. Olympian and the author of a popular series of books on running, believes it isn't actually possible to "listen to the body," as so many coaches recommend, because there are simply too many variables. Reason and logic can't always tell us, for example, why our ankle is hurting, or why we've got less than our usual energy. But intuition—calm feeling—can often deliver the answer.

Intuition works on many levels. Often, it'll be just a simple, earthy feeling about what's right—*Hmm, my body's starting to feel unpleasantly pressed—better slow down.* More rarely, it can express a higher guidance, sometimes in startling ways.

Here's a story of a time when intuition served me well. It's an extreme case, because it touches on intuition's spiritual dimension. But it's not untypical of the intuitive guidance I've received over the years.

I was training for my first ultramarathon, a difficult 50K (31.1-mile) race in the High Sierra with over 9000' of climbing, when Achilles pain threatened to end my running career altogether. I was aware that shoe inserts (orthotics) might help. But money was tight, so I tried everything else I could think of, including anti-inflammatory drugs, motion-control shoes, icing, massage, taping, and cheap over-the-counter inserts. I even stuffed leaves in my shoes! But nothing worked.

Finally, feeling desperate, I inwardly asked my spiritual teacher for guidance. And that's when the answer came, as my teacher's quiet voice: "*Go see the podiatrist.*"

I protested, "But I don't have a lot of money, and the podiatrist will prescribe orthotics that cost $400—plus he'll charge $40 for the office visit."

The inner guidance was unrelenting. Again it said, "*Go see the podiatrist.*" Feeling that I had little to lose, I made the appointment. Sure enough, the podiatrist wanted $40 for the exam and $400 for a set of orthotics. Taking my faith in my hands, I told him to place the order and send me the bill.

The next day, a friend that I hadn't heard from in years called to say that he'd finished writing a book for racing cyclists, and he needed photos. He needed them quickly, and would I do them for $500?

This story has repeated itself, with endless variations, in my 40-plus years as a runner, to the extent that nowadays, whenever I need an answer to a problem with my training, I simply ask. Of course, it isn't *quite* that simple, since getting clear answers takes a certain *kind* of asking and listening, and it's a skill one develops over time.

The answers rarely come in words, as in the story of the podiatrist. More often, it'll be no more than a quiet inner knowing, or a subtle feeling of "rightness" when I try one thing, and an unease when I try the opposite. Other times, I'll be guided to a person, a book, or a series of logical thoughts that hold the answer.

Here's another story from the "intuitive fringe."

This year, I planned to run and fast-hike 52.4 miles, a double marathon, as a fundraiser for a local school.

I was enthusiastic about the route I'd chosen, which started at the north end of the Golden Gate Bridge and wound southward through the neighborhoods of San Francisco, and along the flanks of the Coastal Range to our home in Mountain View.

I've always loved long solo runs, and I'd hauled out my maps and was happily checking distances, when I began to notice an uneasy feeling in my heart.

It was perplexing, because I had covered similar distances in the past. And it was embarrassing, because I had announced my plans to friends. But I couldn't shake the feeling, so I put my plans on hold. When I stopped fretting and got calm, I silently asked if I really shouldn't do the run. And that's when I heard an intuitive voice that said, *"It's too far."*

I swallowed my pride and planned a 35-mile outing instead, on a lovely route from the ocean at Half Moon Bay, over the Coastal Range to the Bay at Mountain View.

During the run, I developed four huge blood blisters that forced me to fast-hike the last 15 miles. Toward the end I could barely shuffle, and I realized that it would have been a disaster to attempt the longer distance. (The good news is that I had a wonderful adventure and raised $1200 for the school.)

I'm certainly not going to claim that my intuition is perfect. But the guidance I receive seems to "work" remarkably well. Intuition has proved itself to my satisfaction in the laboratory of thousands of miles of running.

In the chapters that follow, I'll suggest that all successful and enjoyable training is *expansive*. "Expansion" simply means that we're "stretching our edges" in meaningful ways. We're using the five tools of an athlete—body, heart, will, mind, soul—to create more health, love, strength, wisdom, and joy. When we're able to do that, we feel wonderful, and our training goes well.

But expansion has its dark opposite side. When we use our runner's tools "contractively," we suffer. When we misuse our bodies by overtraining, for example, we shrivel and become less than we were: physically drained, emotionally withdrawn, with little energy for running, work, or relationships.

Sports training is a never-ending battle to do the *right thing*. Winning the battle takes maturity, self-control, and patience. Intuition—the calm and receptive heart—can tell us if we're moving in the right, expansive direction toward greater fitness and joy, or if we're headed in a direction that will lead us into a ditch.

I don't claim that this book will tell you everything there is to know about expansive sports. But I'm confident that these core principles will help you improve your results and create more enjoyable training.

In the chapters that follow, I'll present evidence that expansive attitudes are linked to athletic success at every level. I'll describe the five tools of expansive training, and how nature develops those tools in a natural sequence during the first 24 years of our lives.

We'll discover exciting research that reveals how expansive thoughts and feelings enhance physical performance, mental focus, emotional well-being, intuition, and subjective feelings of being "in touch with Spirit."

In the remaining chapters, I'll suggest that training is evolving away from older mechanistic models, toward energy-based methods that can bring us success and enjoyment more efficiently. As evidence for the validity of expansive sports, I'll present many examples from the experiences of elite athletes and teams.

Sports training holds a promise of experiences of great

depth and joy. It's my hope that this book will contribute to your enjoyment of the athlete's path.

Three Key Principles of Joyful Sports

1. Good training is enjoyable.

2. Enjoyment comes by using the five tools of an athlete expansively: body, heart, will, mind, and soul.

3. Intuition (calm feeling) can help us know what's expansive and will bring us joy, and what's contractive and will stall our progress and kill our enjoyment.

3. THE 5 DIMENSIONS OF FITNESS

I don't read the papers much, but I came across an article in the *Sacramento Bee* several years ago that fairly begged to be disbelieved. Here's an excerpt:

In a *Journal of Medical Ethics* article titled "A Proposal to Classify Happiness as a Psychiatric Disorder," Liverpool University psychologist Richard P. Bentall argues that the so-called syndrome of happiness is a diagnosable mood disturbance that should be included in standard taxonomies of mental illness such as the American Psychiatric Association's Diagnostic and Statistical Manual. Happiness, as Bentall states in his abstract, is "statistically abnormal, consists of a discrete cluster of symptoms, is associated with a range of cognitive abnormalities and probably reflects the abnormal functioning of the central nervous system." (In this regard, as Bentall later notes, happiness resembles other psychiatric disorders such as depression and schizophrenia.)

The author of the *Bee* article, Maggie Scarf, a *New Republic* contributing editor, related Dr. Bentall's suggestion "that the term 'happiness' be removed from future editions of the major diagnostic manuals, to be replaced by the formal description 'major affective disorder, pleasant type.'"

When I read the article aloud to a friend, she promptly doubled over with major affective disorder. "That's such amazing cock-a-doo!" she howled. "It's so carefully reasoned—yet it's completely incredible!"

The Practice of Happiness

It is nutty-cakes. And yet, is there anything actually wrong with using scientific methods to study happiness? After all, it's what the spiritual explorers of all ages have done—studying happiness in the laboratory of their bodies, hearts, and minds, and keeping tidy notes on what works and what doesn't.

For most of us, happiness isn't a "mood disturbance"—it's the answer we're after. And if we can get a bit more with the help of scientific orderliness and method, so much the better.

Because the world's spiritual traditions have made a study of happiness, what they say may be worth hearing in these times of pandemic discontent.

After all, their approach is practical. They tell us, for instance, that we have five instruments through which we can experience happiness: body, heart, will, mind, and soul. And they explain that as we grow into adulthood, we pass through five stages, each lasting six years, during which each of the "tools," in the order I've listed them, becomes the primary developmental focus.

Happiness, they say, increases when we learn to use each tool "expansively." (More on expansion later.) Thus, the most important time in our lives for learning to be happy is when we're growing up, passing through the six-year stages.

From birth to age 6, an infant's primary developmental focus is on becoming familiar with its body and senses. From 6 to 12, the child's feelings come to the fore—it's a time when children are particularly receptive to learning through the arts—the "media of feeling," including stories, music, theater, art, and dance.

From 12 to 18, teenagers embrace challenges to their will power in preparation for independent adult life. And at around 18, young people become fascinated with the life of the mind, engaging in discussions of politics, science, the arts, and philosophy.

Finally, at about age 24, many people experience major life events that may precede a spiritual awakening.

As each tool takes center stage, the others don't simply fade away. Thus, while a toddler is primarily concerned with its body and senses, it doesn't hesitate to express its feelings—with the volume turned up! Nor do the stages begin exactly on our 6th, 12th, 18th, and 24th birthdays; the transitions are gradual.

Why did nature settle on this particular scheme? In his insightful book, *Education for Life*, J. Donald Walters explains how each stage prepares the child for the ones that follow. Thus, feeling comes before will power, because feeling is the faculty that enables us to tell right from wrong. Before we can use our will power appropriately, with awareness of others, we need to develop the ability to *feel* their realities. Walters laments the ruinous consequences of cramming children's minds with facts, at the expense of developing their capacity to feel sensitively, as is common in schools today.

Similarly, each stage fulfills the preceding one. Thus, feeling motivates us to action, and will power provides the energy and focus to act on our feelings. Unless we *want* something strongly enough, we won't exert the energy to achieve it.

Will power, in turn, finds its fulfillment in wisdom, which tells us which actions will make us happy and which won't. And wisdom is fulfilled in Spirit. In Self-realization, we realize that all wisdom and joy come from an ultimate Source within.

The history of education reveals that in ancient Greece and Rome, and throughout the Middle Ages and Enlightenment, the six-year stages were recognized as natural phases of a child's growth. Thus appropriate teaching methods were devised for each stage, and schools were roughly divided into the equivalents of our modern elementary school (ages 6–12), junior and senior high (12–18), and college (18–24).

Expanding Awareness Equals Joy

As I hinted earlier, the spiritual teachings of the ages tell us that happiness increases as we learn to use our five human tools "expansively." Like most abstractions, "expansion" is easiest to understand with examples. At the risk of repetition, let's look at what happens when we begin an exercise program, as we did in the last chapter.

After the first two or three weeks, we find that we're feeling happier and more alive. Why? Because the exercising body has begun to generate energy, which spills over to nourish our feelings, will, and mind, expanding their range and force. Expanding our awareness through one "tool," the body, influences the others. Good actions spread their effects—as do "bad" ones.

The spiritual researchers of all ages and cultures realized that the single underlying desire that drives all our actions is a longing to experience greater happiness, and to escape from sorrow.

Albert Einstein, ever a perceptive observer of the human scene, stated it this way:

> Everything that the human race has done and thought is concerned with the satisfaction of deeply felt needs and

the assuagement of pain. One has to keep this constantly in mind if one wishes to understand spiritual movements and their development. Feeling and longing are the motive force behind all human endeavor and human creation, in however exalted a guise the latter may present themselves. (From the essay, "Cosmic Religious Feeling.")

People tend to specialize in one, or perhaps two, of the "tools of expansion." Thus, some people go more by feeling, while others tend to "lead" with their willpower or mind. The spiritual teachings encourage us to go with our strengths, while working to correct any imbalances.

It's fascinating to watch runners with a view to identifying their primary "tool" from their running style. Some runners "lead with their hearts"—chest out, smiling and confident. Others lead with their minds, heads thrust forward or lowered in thought, while others go more by willpower, bulling their way with their foreheads, as if to blast away obstacles.

In many natural processes, the "tools of happiness" tend to appear in the same sequence as in a child's development. When we fall in love, for example, the first attraction is most often, though not always, physical. We see a person across the room whose appearance attracts us, and our feelings become aroused. We form a volition to act on our feelings, and we walk over and strike up a conversation. The mind probes for information: *Is she married? Does he like children?* And if we're wise, we'll consult a higher guidance before entering this potential new life venture. We've passed through the five "tools" in order: body, feeling, will, mind, soul.

When I ran ultramarathons, I noticed that the tools tended to show up in the same order. The first hour or two were for the body, as I found my rhythm and my body began to generate a flow of energy. The next hour was for the heart

—cheerful conversations often sprang up among the runners. As my body tired, willpower came to the fore—it was time to gather my forces and not waste energy on distractions.

Farther along, it became important to apply the mind to questions of logistics: How can I fuel my body and pace myself to make it to the next aid station? How can I deal with this blister?

Finally, if I succeeded in using the tools well, I would enjoy a wonderful inner freedom. I became a very simple person, free from distractions, worries, and restless thoughts, living wholly in the moment.

Talking with other runners, I found that they'd experienced a similar sequence in the longer rhythms of their careers.

At the start, the major issues tended to be about the body—how to train, which shoes to wear, how to treat an injury, what to eat and drink, etc.

Later, as the body grew fit, feelings came front and center. The feeling stage is rich with the romance of running, as we explore longer distances, seek challenging courses, and absorb the inspiration of successful runners.

Later, we crave challenges to our will. We might take up speedwork and enter more difficult races. As we pass through the five phases, we discover that the tools we need for the next stage tend to show up in uncanny ways.

After the willpower phase, runners often become intrigued by the life of the mind. They learn to plan their training carefully, perhaps using a heart monitor.

Finally, there may be a period where the overriding concerns are spiritual, and all of the tools are merged in a quest for inner harmony. We seek a fulfillment that comes when we "run in beauty," our activities balanced in careful synchrony.

It helps to be aware of the five stages of a run, and the natural sequence of a runner's career. It can help us make appropriate decisions at each stage, deliberately focusing on the "tool of the moment" as we prepare for the stage that follows.

More than we tend to realize, each of the tools is a world unto itself, with unique strengths and rewards.

In my life, I've had the good fortune to enter two of these worlds as a relative newcomer. First, when I started an exercise program, and later when I spent several years working to open my heart.

In the first case, I was amazed to discover the world of the fit body. I had never been in shape, and now, at age 26, I could run for miles barefoot on the beach, probing with fingers of consciousness into the rich inner world of a body that glowed with health and energy. How fulfilling and expansive it was, to enter this spacious new world for the first time!

Later, as my heart began to open, I was delighted to discover the vast inner world of feeling. I became aware that there were issues in my life for which the heart held answers that were hidden to the rational mind. I learned to appreciate the world of feeling in which women spend much of their lives. Standing in line at the bank or supermarket, I could enjoy watching women working together, appreciating their communion of feeling.

The System Is Rigged

It all sounds so simple and straightforward—just use the tools expansively and happiness will follow, rather like remembering to brush our teeth in the morning. But in real life, cultivating expansive attitudes turns out to be a challenge. That's because, as I mentioned earlier, the opposite urge, contraction, is strong in us also.

Life places essentially the same choice continually before us: will we use our bodies wisely, or abuse them? Our hearts, to love or to hate? Our minds, to be wise or merely clever? Our spiritual instincts, to aspire or to dabble in psychic trivialities? History—ours and the world's—is the story of the eternal struggle between these opposing forces in human nature.

Also, the theory is simple, but the details aren't. We've been given all the tools we require to achieve happiness and success—or so it seems. The trouble is, relying too exclusively on our purely human toolbox, we find ourselves sooner or later bumping against its limitations.

The five tools of expansion embody wonderful expertise, yet their very specialization can trip us. When this happens, we can still find answers by looking beyond the tools. Happily, we can use these same instruments to tap into an awareness that is fathomlessly wise and loving, and that has our best interests at heart.

That's what expansive sports is about: using our intuition to fine-tune our training for success and joy.

But what of Professor Bentall? Researchers are discovering that, for athletes and everyone, happiness is good medicine. I'll review some of these findings in chapter 5 ("Science of the Heart").

4. THE HARMONY ZONE

Many years ago, I began to notice that my runs tended to be more enjoyable when I warmed up at a specific pace.

There was a feeling of harmony and "rightness" that came when I started my runs at that pace. It was a subtle feeling in my heart, a bare, faint whisper that grew stronger if I ran as those inner feelings directed.

It took me years to begin to trust those undertones of feeling. At first they were so subtle that I brushed them impatiently aside. It was a tiny flicker in my heart, and although it never actually *told* me what to do, I sensed that it was quietly suggesting what my body *could* do healthily, or "wanted" to do, on a given day.

The problem was that it often sent messages I didn't want to hear. My training motto at the time was "everything to excess, nothing in moderation." I enjoyed the extremes of running—the hard speedwork and long runs—and when I began to hear the messages from my heart, they often seemed to be telling me to run more moderately.

I thought, "Well, that's interesting, and maybe those feelings are right. But they don't jibe with the latest research, or the advice of great coaches. Anyway, I just don't feel like running slowly today!" So I ignored them. Yet over the ensuing years, I gradually realized that whenever I paid attention and followed the inner guidance—or when I was so battered and bruised from overtraining that I had no choice—my runs were more enjoyable and I made better progress. Thus I slowly, reluctantly, came to respect the wisdom of the heart.

In time, I learned of coaches whose methods were in sync with my own experiences. They were people like Arthur Lydiard, Philip Maffetone, and John Douillard, whose ideas were sometimes far removed from the coaching mainstream, but had been tested at the highest competitive levels.

Year after year, professional triathlete Mark Allen failed to win the Hawaii Ironman Triathlon. After hiring Phil Maffetone as his coach, he won the Ironman six times.

Intrigued by Allen's success, short-course triathlon world champion Mike Pigg consulted Maffetone and experienced similar improvements. Another Maffetone client was Priscilla Welch, the women's master's marathon world record holder (2:26:51 at age 41, London, 1987).

John Douillard is a former professional triathlete whose coaching clients included world-champion short-course triathlete Colleen Cannon. Douillard's methods have been used with success by high-school cross-country teams and many individual runners.

Although the details of their programs differ, the Maffetone and Douillard systems are consistent with the "harmony-zone" principle I discovered by listening to my heart. Yet the messages I receive when I'm running in the harmony zone can't really be confined to a system. They aren't a system, but a method for getting the best from *any* system, by adjusting it to our own body's unique, ever-changing needs.

Occasionally those inner signals will give us "permission" to do things that contradict any fixed training plan—like breaking out of the box and running faster or farther than the schedule calls for. When those "outlaw" runs have the backing of the intuitive heart, we come out of them feeling wonderful.

I suspect that for most runners, training in the harmony zone won't come easily. It's an exacting discipline, because it demands a commitment to do whatever the heart "wants," even if it means jogging slowly when the body isn't ready for anything faster.

What's the best training pace for entering the harmony zone? There's no clear-cut answer. For a long time, my personal "harmony zone" pace seemed to hover between 70–78% of my maximum heart rate. It might be higher or lower on a given day, depending on recovery, diet, the weather, etc.

Later, I realized that the feelings of harmony seemed to be strongest at 77–78% of MHR. Still later, I discovered that on long runs, the harmony zone was generally lower, around 70%.

To confuse matters, I would occasionally have those feelings of "rightness" while running at a *very* fast pace, above 90% MHR.

I was baffled. How could there be so many harmony zones? In time, I realized the obvious answer: there is no single "best" zone or heart rate. The feelings of harmony on a particular day were my body's guide to what it could safely and happily do. If I ran at the speed and distance my heart allowed, I was rewarded with enjoyable feelings and improving fitness.

One thing was consistent: the harmony zone pace was nearly always much slower at the start of a run. Also, it struck me that I *never* got those good feelings if my body wasn't fully recovered—if its message was *"Help! I'm trashed! Take me home!"*

On the days when I was deeply tired, or mildly ill, I might

experience the good feelings for a few miles, but if I went farther or picked up the pace, they would vanish. Often, they would return if I slowed down.

Those feelings always grew stronger when I "did the right thing." From these experiences, I realized that the harmony zone is more than a strictly mechanical "feedback loop" between my body and mind. The feelings in my heart expressed a deep interior wisdom that was mindful of my overall well-being. When I ran in the harmony state, there was a wholesome sense of health and happiness, and I more often had runs where my body, heart, and mind seemed beautifully synchronized.

Finding the harmony zone became an enjoyable preamble to each run. No mystical mumbo-jumbo was required, nor much rational thought. Yet a variety of wonderful experiences grew out of that simple, earthy attunement that began with the warmup.

As I explored the harmony zone, I discovered that I could deepen the experience by deliberately cultivating positive feelings. It wasn't a question of *thinking* my way into a better mood, but of using "heart means" to amplify any positive sensations that were already present. Too much thinking just seemed to get in the way.

One "heart method" that worked well was silently sending good thoughts to the people I encountered on the trail. Or I might take a phrase that held positive associations for me and repeat it silently. It might be a few lines from a song, or an affirmation, a chant, or a prayer. If I couldn't find anything to "wrap my heart around," it often worked best just to cultivate a smooth, harmonious flow of energy.

If I've learned one thing as a runner, it's that good feelings and good training go together. The best training produces steady improvement and an upbeat mood. Runs that "feel bad" usually result in failure to improve. Frank Shorter said he felt that runners get more out of their training when they run in places where they feel happy and at ease. I believe it's worth a lot to find those places, even if it takes some extra gas to get there.

Many years ago, I experienced the harmony zone in a particularly striking way, during a 20-mile run in the foothills of the San Francisco Peninsula. Halfway into the run, my tank was empty. I was miles from anywhere and didn't want to walk home, so I kept plodding.

I wore a heart monitor, and I noticed that if I tried to hold my heart rate at the planned 78% pace, I felt stressed and strained, but when I slowed to 72% I felt—and this is what surprised me—wonderful, even though I had crashed badly.

That run lingers in memory as one of my best. Why? Because I paid attention to what my body was telling me. I listened to my heart and ran as it suggested, and my body-mind-soul rewarded me.

Seventeen miles into the run, I was climbing the last hill, jogging on a sidewalk by a street with heavy traffic. The hill was long and steep, and I had to slow to a shuffle to keep my heart rate down and preserve the feelings of rightness. I'm not a fan of shuffling, but I was feeling so wonderful that I couldn't refrain from singing aloud. That run gave me all the proof I would ever need that the quiet joy in my heart is a reliable guide for my training.

I can't explain the harmony zone rationally, except to imagine that the heart is the loudspeaker for a higher wisdom in the brain, or perhaps the soul. It's as if our body, heart, and brain intuitively know: "We'll be running 20 miles today. If we go at Y pace we'll feel fine, but if we go any faster, we'll crash."

Several years ago, I asked Timothy Noakes, MD, the author of *Lore of Running*, for his thoughts on some ideas I wanted to include in this book. Here's how Dr. Noakes answered in an email:

> In the new [fourth] edition of *Lore of Running* you will see that our new research suggests that the major effect of training is to induce a superior pacing strategy which is determined centrally in the brain. We now believe that the brain controls performance, not the muscles, although with training, the increase in aerobic enzyme activities tells the brain that the body is capable of more. However, the principal determinant of performance remains the adaptations in the brain which must be fooled (or trained—you choose the appropriate verb) to allow you to run faster than it would normally allow.
>
> I understand that this sounds like a foreign language, but the evidence we have is absolutely clear; the brain is in charge, and it decides when to reduce your speed as you get tired, and [the evidence also suggests] that this reduction in pace probably is in response to numerous stimuli coming from the muscles and other parts of the body. However, it is the subconscious brain that chooses the pace that it will allow you to do, and it always chooses a pace that will ensure you do not collapse or die before the finish of the race. The very fact that there is this safety factor indicates that the brain is ultimately in charge.

These views were confirmed in later research by a colleague of Noakes's at the University of Cape Town:

> Traditionally, fatigue was viewed as the result of over-worked muscles ceasing to function properly. But evidence is mounting that our brains make us feel weary

after exercise. . . . The idea is that the brain steps in to prevent muscle damage.

Now Paula Robson-Ansley and her colleagues at the University of Cape Town in South Africa have demonstrated that a ubiquitous body signalling molecule called interleukin-6 plays a key role in telling the brain when to slow us down. Blood levels of IL-6 are 60 to 100 times higher than normal following prolonged exercise, and injecting healthy people with IL-6 makes them feel tired.

To work out if IL-6 affects performance, Robson-Ansley injected seven club-standard runners with either IL-6 or a placebo and recorded their times over 10 kilometres. A week later, the experiment was reversed.

On average they ran nearly a minute faster after receiving the placebo, a significant difference since their finishing times were around 41 minutes. The findings will appear in the *Canadian Journal of Applied Physiology*.[10]

Our rational, logical minds can help us understand how to train, given adequate data. But when the data are lacking or deeply hidden, we can augment our decision-making ability with intuition—by tapping a stream of *inner* data that the body communicates to us through our feelings.

One of America's greatest middle-distance runners, Bob Kennedy, is aware of the need to go "beyond the brain" in training. The first American to run 5000 meters in under 13 minutes, Bob says feelings are a valuable ally:

[Interviewer:] What about the idea of pushing oneself in a good way, versus pushing too far. How do you tell

---

10. "Brain not body makes athletes feel tired," Newscientist.com, July 29, 2004. http://www.newscientist.com/article.ns?id=dn6208. Downloaded on May 6, 2005.

the difference between challenging yourself and going overboard?

Bob Kennedy: You have to really pay attention to your body, not only physically, but mentally and emotionally. As soon as you start not enjoying what you're doing—or start really struggling and go for a run and think "what am I doing out here"—if that starts becoming the norm, then you're pushing too hard and something's not right. You know, back off, take a rest, or reorganize yourself. But if you're pushing hard and doing some speed and some longer runs, and you're really fired up about it, and you're giving yourself some recovery time, then you know you're pushing yourself in a good way.[11]

World-champion age-group Olympic weightlifters Jerzy and Aniela Gregorek write:

The slogan "No pain, no gain" characterizes bad coaches and ignorant athletes. . . . Intelligent weightlifters learn to follow the signs given by the body. They analyze every feeling to adjust training daily to ensure recovery and smooth progress."[12]

Birdwatchers have a saying, "When the bird and the book disagree, believe the bird." The heart's intuitive feelings can be a valuable addition to our athlete's toolbox, one we've neglected for too long in our reason-addicted culture.

---

11.   Downloaded   from   http://www.nike.com/nikerunning/usa/home. jhtml?ref=http://www.nike.com/nikerunning#runners_library on July 1, 2005 at 12:22 PDT.

12. Downloaded on September 12, 2005 from: http://www.thehappybody.com/ Seminars/San%20Francisco%20Bay.pdf.

5. SCIENCE OF THE HEART

Scientists at HeartMath Research Center in Boulder Creek, California, are studying the effects of positive feelings such as love, compassion, and kindness on our bodies and brains. Their research supports the notion that it's important for athletes to "accentuate the positive, eliminate the negative, and don't mess with Mister In-Between."[13]

(Disclaimer: I have no financial or other business interest in HeartMath or its products.)

Here are some of the HeartMath findings:

- Positive emotional states exert a whole-body synchronizing effect by bringing brain waves, heart rhythms, breathing, and blood-pressure oscillations into a unified, harmonious rhythm. During positive feelings, "bodily systems function with a high degree of synchronization, efficiency and harmony."

- Deliberately focusing attention in the heart while cultivating feelings of love, compassion, etc., leads to clearer thinking, calmer emotions, and improved physical performance and health, as well as increased frequency of subjective reports of spiritual experiences.

- Positive, expansive feelings such as love, appreciation,

---

13. The basic HeartMath research is described in *The HeartMath Solution* by Doc Childre and Howard Martin (HarperSanFrancisco, 1999), as well as in research papers on the organization's website, www.heartmath.org.

and compassion promote relaxation and synchronization of the nervous system. They quiet the "arousal" (sympathetic) branch of the nervous system and activate the "relaxation" (parasympathetic) side. The sympathetic branch of the autonomic nervous system is responsible for speeding up heart rate and preparing the body for action, while the parasympathetic branch governs the "relaxation response," slowing heart rate and calming body, emotions, and brain.

- Positive feelings quiet the mind, generate a sense of "self-security, peace and love," and increase the frequency of reported feelings of "connectedness to God."
- Additionally, the researchers found that negative emotions such as anger, fear, and hatred make the heartbeat change speeds erratically—the heart literally speeds up and slows down chaotically from one beat to the next, like the random, jerky motion of a car that's running out of gas. (See figure below.)

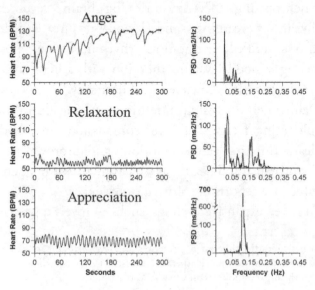

- Positive emotions such as love, compassion, and appreciation, on the other hand, make the heart beat with a harmonious, regular rhythm. During negative emotions, the heart's irregular speed-changes appear as jagged, disordered spikes, and its power output is relatively low. Simple relaxation produces a more regular rhythm. But deliberately cultivating positive emotions makes the heart beat in a steady, consistent, harmonious rhythm, reflected in the regular, sine-wave-like pattern in the figure ("Appreciation"). During positive emotions, the heart's power output jumps by over 500% above the levels attained during negative emotions and simple relaxation. (In the figure, note the Power Spectral Density [PSD] scale in "Appreciation.") The coherent mode doesn't appear to depend on heart rate; coherency can appear at high or low heart rates—i.e., harmonious feelings and heart-brain-body synchronization can occur at any running speed.

The HeartMath findings have begun to find practical applications in professional sports. Here's an excerpt from an article on the website of the Professional Golfers' Association (PGA):

When we're stressed or upset, it's physically impossible to think clearly or perform at our best. This is because a disordered heart rhythm pattern sends a signal to the brain that inhibits the cortex, the higher thinking and reasoning part of the brain. On the other hand, when we are feeling confident, secure, and appreciative, our heart rhythms become smooth and even. . . . Smooth heart rhythm patterns send a signal to the brain that synchronizes and facilitates cortical function, speeding up our reaction times and making it easier to think clearly, perceive a bigger picture, and make better decisions.[14]

The heart and brain communicate continually through the nervous system. Thus the heart's powerful positive or negative, harmonizing or disruptive messages are carried instantly to the brain, where they enhance or interfere with our ability to remain cool and concentrate. (The heart is the body's most powerful oscillator, sending out electrical signals roughly 60 times as strong those emitted by the brain.)

To summarize: positive, harmonious feelings enhance mental focus, calmness, health, performance, intuition (as we'll see shortly), and the frequency of spiritual feelings. They increase relaxation, alpha-wave output in the brain (associated with a calm, meditative state), and synchronize heart-rhythm patterns, respiratory rhythms, and blood pressure oscillations.

Whether our goal is peak performance, "inner quality," zone experiences, or spiritual communion, it's good to remember that changing our feelings can be a powerful aid. Anything we can do to stimulate positive feelings, including running in the harmony zone, will assist clear thinking and boost physical performance.

The HeartMath scientists have also discovered that the rhythms of a person's heart may synchronize with another person's heartbeat at distances up to five feet—good reason to keep company with positive, upbeat people, and to avoid whiners and complainers.

As athletes, we have a special advantage. On days when it's difficult to muster positive feelings, we can "work the other way round," and use our bodies to stimulate a buoyant

---

14. Deborah Rozman, PhD, Pia Nilsson, and Lynn Marriott, "Second That Emotion," downloaded from www.pga.com in 2004. *Gold Digest* readers voted Pia Nilsson and Lynn Marriott to the magazine's list of the top 50 US golf coaches.

mood. Many spiritual traditions recommend rhythmic movement—dancing, running, physical postures, etc.—to harmonize and uplift our physical energy and heal our hearts and minds.

Focusing attention and energy in the area of the *physical* heart, while dwelling on positive thoughts, feelings, and memories, is one effective approach to achieving "psychophysiological coherence." Breathing exercises are another.

In *Body, Mind, and Sport,* former professional triathlete John Douillard, mentioned earlier, describes a breathing technique that increases oxygen absorption in the lungs and stimulates parasympathetic (relaxation) nerve centers in the lower lungs. Douillard's field tests showed that the method also increases alpha-wave production in the brain, indicative of a meditative, zone-like state.

Douillard borrowed the breathing technique from yoga. In yoga lore, it's believed that it stimulates the prefrontal cortex, the brain area where certain positive attitudes and abilities are localized, such as mental focus, optimism, and the ability to create and persevere in attaining long-term goals.

The method involves nose-breathing, while optionally making a "Darth Vader" sound in the throat during exhalation, as if you were blowing on a pair of glasses— "Aaah"—but with your mouth closed. Don't laugh—it may take several weeks to get used to nose-breathing, but it does work. Douillard explains that in all mammals, mouth-breathing is associated with a fight-or-flight response, while nose-breathing is associated with calmness and poise. During training runs of up to 35 miles, I've found that I'm more relaxed, focused, and less tired when I nose-breathe, though I rarely practice the Darth Vader sound. May the Force be with you.

Several high-end Polar heart monitors use heart-rate variability data to help runners determine their best individual warmup pace. At the start of a run, the amplitude of heart-rate variability falls off rapidly until a runner's heart rate reaches roughly 65% of maximum, whereupon the amplitude levels off and falls much more gradually as running speed increases. The Polar monitors signal a runner when their heart rate reaches the 65% plateau. The Polar scientists feel this is a safer, more precise way to determine a sensible 65% warmup pace than testing maximum heart rate with a stressful all-out run, or using notoriously inaccurate age-based formulas and tables. You simply start running slowly and let the monitor tell you when you've reached 65% of your max heart rate.

It's important to note that the initial fall-off in amplitude of heart-rate variability doesn't indicate that running, by itself, reduces heart-rate variability, or that faster running makes us feel calmer and more positive. What happens is that, as the heart beats faster, there's less time for large variations in heart rate to develop. Think of it this way: when your feelings are negative, your heart still changes speed chaotically, but with a faster, lighter beat if you run faster.

John Douillard recommends warming up no faster than approximately 50% of maximum heart rate, calculated by the Karvonen formula (for me, though of course not for everyone, this works out to just under 65% of MHR). To calculate 50% of your MHR by the Karvonen formula, subtract your resting heart rate from your maximum heart rate; divide the resulting number by 2, than add your resting heart rate.

In his book, Douillard reports that Kenneth Cooper, the Aerobics pioneer, now suggests that the optimal pace for general fitness running is about 65% of maximum heart rate (as a straight percentage of MHR, not by the Karvonen formula).

What's certain is that positive feelings help our hearts and bodies work more efficiently, whether we're jogging at aerobic pace or racing an all-out 5K.

6. FOCUS ON FEELING

On a summer afternoon many years ago, I was running trails in the Sierra foothills when I noticed that I'd fallen into a deeply harmonious state. I realized that my breathing was perfectly synchronized with my footfall—I don't recall the pattern; perhaps it was three or four footsteps per breath.

I thought, "I wonder if my breathing and footfall are also in sync with my heartbeat."

I stopped and checked my pulse, then resumed running and stopped several more times and repeated the experiment. Sure enough, my breathing, footfall, and heartbeat were "oscillating" in perfect rhythm.

Researchers at HeartMath Institute have devised exercises that help people deliberately cultivate "coherent" states such as I experienced on that long-ago summer day. For example, "Freeze-Framing" involves taking a deliberate time-out from negative emotions, while holding attention in the area of the heart and dwelling deeply on the memory of an experience of love, compassion, or some other positive feeling. Freeze-Framing and other HeartMath methods have helped children perform better in school. They've served as effective stress-busters for police, business executives, and others in high-wire jobs.

Could anyone have predicted that the Professional Golfers' Association (PGA), one of the most conservative governing bodies in sports, would host articles on its website with titles like "Appreciation and Compassion," and "Recouping Emotional Energy"? (www.pga.com) The articles were co-authored by leading PGA teaching professionals together with Deborah Rozman, PhD, president of Quantum Intech, Inc. (www.quantumintech.com), a company that develops products and services based on the HeartMath research.

An interesting Quantum Intech gadget is the Freeze-Framer, a device that connects to a desktop computer and reads heart-rate variability patterns from the subject's finger pulse. These patterns are displayed on the PC screen, where they provide feedback for video game-like exercises that help the subject learn to create the coherent state at will.

A HeartMath technique that's free, and can be practiced anywhere, is "Quick Coherence." Rozman and Laird Small, the PGA's 2003 Teacher of the Year, described it in an article on the PGA website, "Managing Emotions—The Zone":

Briefly, you focus your attention on your heart, then breathe as if you're breathing through your heart slowly for a few seconds, then find something to feel appreciation for while you're breathing through the heart. It's the positive feeling for what you're appreciating (not the thoughts about it) synchronized with heart breathing that creates coherence. You can watch how this works if you practice Quick Coherence with the Freeze-Framer heart rhythm monitor and see your heart rhythms change into a smooth and coherent pattern as your emotions and attitude change.

On the run, it takes only a little practice to find your personal harmony zone. Try starting the run at a slow pace, where the harmony zone tends to occur more easily during the warmup—say, 65% of maximum heart rate. Or you might try warming up at about 50% of maximum heart rate calculated by the Karvonen formula (maximum heart rate minus resting heart rate, divided by 2, plus resting heart rate).

No need to be overly technical—the 65%/50% guideline is a starting point for personal experimentation. The idea is to run relaxed and easy, at a pace that feels comfortable and natural, where your breathing is deep and slow.

Another easy way to locate your best warmup pace is by "listening" to the feelings of your heart. Start slowly, and as your pace increases, "watch" your heart. At the point where you begin to feel the slightest disharmony or discomfort, back off and run a little slower. Those feelings of discomfort are the body's subtle way of letting you know it isn't ready to run faster. When the body is fully warmed up—assuming you're fit, rested, and not ill—you'll no longer feel those discordant sensations when you bump up the pace.

On some days, following a long warmup, you'll be able to run very hard without any discomfort at all. (See chapter 46, "The 96% Run.") Bear in mind, the heart's feelings will seldom *order* you to run fast—that decision is up to you. But the heart will let you know when it's *okay*—safe and healthy— to put the pedal to the metal. Your intuition may occasionally even suggest a faster warmup pace—or no warmup at all. I suspect this happens when, for reasons we may not be clearly aware of, it's in our best interests to do some fast running— perhaps to break out of physical staleness, a negative mood, or the emotional blahs.

This morning, a friend dropped me off at the bank on her way to work. I made my deposit and began walking home. I've been recovering from a 35-mile run/hike for our school's jogathon. I got bad blisters during the event, and it's been a week since I've run. As I walked, I sensed my body was eager to run, and I took off at a blistering pace, full of the joy of running. No big warmup, no deliberate, careful preparation (though I did listen for a silent "okay" in my heart).

I ran two hard sprints of 200–400 yards, and it felt terrific—there wasn't the slightest feeling of inner resistance, "wrongness," or disharmony. I suspect the higher intelligence sometimes just wants to cut loose and *fly!*

On days when your body is ill, tired, or stressed, your harmony zone may remain quite low. The best way I know to tell if you've truly been running in the harmony zone is how you feel *after*. Running the way the body "wants" nearly always generates good feelings.

It may be hard to hold a slow pace, on days when the body announces it just wants to loaf. But the heart knows.

Occasional slow days are a small price to pay for steadily improving fitness, and the option to do runs of very high quality. On the slow days, I find it helps to remember that Frank Shorter ran all but about 20% of his weekly 140 miles at around 7:00 pace, which for him was very easy. (Shorter's marathon pace was 4:59.)

Another way to locate your harmony zone is by watching your breath. If you're breathing slowly and evenly, and if there's a pause at the end of each out-breath, you're probably running at a pace that's compatible with the harmony zone.

If you're well-trained, you may find that after a thorough warmup your breathing slows noticeably, even as your pace increases. You may have had the strange experience, near the end of a long run, of barely breathing at all while you sailed along at a fast clip.

A heart monitor can help you get a feeling for the harmony zone. The monitor will keep you honest. But over time, the most reliable gauge is the subjective feelings of the heart.

At one point, I tried relying a hundred percent on intuitive feeling to guide my training, but after several months I had to concede that the experiment was a bust. My training was a shambles—I was often overtrained, and I could seldom feel exactly how fast or far my body was prepared to run. I wondered if my intuition simply wasn't well-developed enough to serve as a guide.

I realized that intuition needs to be balanced with common sense. In fact, there's solid scientific evidence that feeling and reason work together, and that relying on one without the other is unwise.

Roughly 70 years ago, researchers became aware that the brain's prefrontal cortex is the "control center," where calm, positive feelings are localized and raw emotions are restrained and modulated. In some spiritual paths, a primary meditative practice involves holding attention gently in the prefrontal cortex, at the point between the eyebrows, a technique those traditions claim has a powerful harmonizing effect on the emotions, and calms and focuses the mind.

In his bestselling book, *Emotional Intelligence, New York Times* science reporter Daniel Goleman relates how the pioneering Russian neuropsychologist A. R. Luria suggested that the prefrontal cortex was a key brain center for self-control and restraining emotional impulses. Luria found that patients with damage to this area "were impulsive and prone to flare-ups of fear and anger."

A study of two dozen men and women convicted of heat-of-passion murders "found . . . that they had a much lower than usual level of activity in these same sections of the prefrontal cortex."[15]

---

15. Daniel Goldman, *Emotional Intelligence.* (New York: Bantam Books, 1995), 314.

In 2002, scientists at Duke University used brain scans to verify that raw emotions interfere with concentration, and that mental focus and emotion exist in a *mutually exclusive* relationship. That is, not only does emotion distort our ability to focus, but deliberately focusing attention is an effective way to calm and "neutralize" raw emotions. As the Duke news release put it, "Surprisingly, an increase in one type of function is accompanied by a noticeable decrease in the other."

This is interesting news for athletes. It's especially relevant for competitors, since it confirms the age-old maxim that deliberately focusing attention tends to calm the pre-race jitters, while uncontrolled emotions are dangerous, because they can interfere with concentration and good decision-making.

Consider the experiences of two runners at the 2002 US Olympic Trials:

Everyone gets nervous before races. "If you're not nervous, you're not excited," says U.S. 5,000m Olympian Brad Hauser. But poorly managed pre-race anxiety can undo months of training by misdirecting your energies away from the task at hand—racing your best. Case in point: Hauser's fifth-place finish in the 10,000m trials. "I made a rookie mistake," admits Hauser. "I was too excited. When the running got hard I was too focused on the result, on making the team."

Nick Rogers, who finished third in the 5,000m after a DNF at 10K, admits, "Anxiety is the reason I didn't make the 10K team. I knew I was one of the top contenders and I just let the pressure get to me. I didn't have fun. For me, anxiety can make me almost focus too much on the race."[16]

Distracting emotions led Hauser and Rose to worry about results, instead of calmly focusing in the moment, on running their best race.

Deliberately focusing attention in the prefrontal cortex can help the mind become relaxed and one-pointed—an asset for runners who want to race well, or simply improve the quality of their runs.

"We've known for a long time that some people are more easily distracted and that emotions can play a big part in this," said Kevin S. LaBarr, assistant professor at Duke's Center for Cognitive Neuroscience and an author of the [above-mentioned] study. "Our study shows that two streams of processing take place in the brain, with attentional tasks and emotions moving in parallel before finally coming together." The two streams are integrated in a region of the brain called the anterior cingulate, which is located between the right and left halves of the brain's frontal portion and is involved in a wide range of thought processes and emotional responses.[17]

I find that holding my attention persistently, with deep relaxation, in the area of the anterior cingulate (behind the point between the eyebrows) helps soothe any troubling emotions I might be feeling, and helps me become more calm, positive, and concentrated.

In fact, researchers now suspect that feeling and reason work hand in hand. Contrary to a longstanding prejudice of our Western culture, which assumes that reason is the superior faculty, researchers are finding that reason is deeply

16. Reproduced by permission. Gordon Bloch, "Nervous—Who Me?" *Running Times*, November 2000, 63. © 2000 Running Times. www.runningtimes.com.

17. Duke University press release, August 19, 2002.

compromised unless it's balanced by the feelings of the heart.

Neurologist Dr. Antonio Damasio studied patients with damage to the connection between their brain's prefrontal cortex and amygdale – the main link between important these two emotional and reasoning centers of the brain. He found that when these patients lost their ability feel, they made terrible decisions in their business and personal lives, and became incapable of making the simplest decisions such as when to make an appointment, even though their reasoning powers were intact.

Dr. Damasio believes their decisions are so bad because they have lost access to their *emotional* learning. . . . Cut off from emotional memory in the amygdala, whatever the neocortex mulls over no longer triggers the emotional reactions that have been associated with it in the past— everything takes on a gray neutrality. . . .

Evidence like this leads Dr. Damasio to the counter-intuitive position that feelings are typically *indispensable* for rational decisions; they point us in the proper direction, where dry logic can then be of best use.[18]

Economists have begun to study how people's brain scans reflect their financial decisions. Their brain waves indicate whether their decision-making is based on calm, clear reason or emotional factors. An article in *BusinessWeek Online* described the research:

For decisions about the far-off future, the prefrontal cortex takes a long-term perspective. But for decisions such as whether to buy another chocolate bar right now, the limbic system takes over and demands immediate gratification. Last year the journal *Science* published the

---

18. Daniel Goleman, *Emotional Intelligence* (New York: Bantam Books, 1997), 27–28.

research by [Harvard University economist David I.] Laibson, Princeton University neuroscientists Samuel M. McClure and Jonathan D. Cohen, and Carnegie-Mellon University economist George Loewenstein. . . .

Even believers in neuroeconomics aren't sure just how far to take it. Should economic policy satisfy the farsighted prefrontal cortex? Or should it sometimes indulge the impulsive limbic system? By peering into the brain, economists are making discoveries that will keep them arguing for years to come.[19]

When I tried training purely by feeling and intuition, my decisions were often prejudiced by my personal desires and emotions. My heart wasn't sufficiently calm and detached to be trusted.

My feelings were more reliable when I checked them against my reason, common sense, and experience. Were my heart's feelings *truly* calm and dispassionate? Or was I just telling myself what I wanted to hear? Was I actually listening to a higher guidance, or was I tuned to some lower, more personal frequency? Cool, clear *reason* helped me decide. My sense of the right training was more often correct when I held myself in a state of "reasonable feeling." It helped to imagine that I was centered in an axis of energy between the forehead and the heart.

During my deepest intuitive experiences, there was a powerful sense of the physical centers of reason and feeling being activated at the same time. My attention was strongly focused, with a sensation of energy gathered in my forehead, in the prefrontal cortex where concentration is localized, but

---

19. *BusinessWeek* Online, March 28, 2005. Downloaded from http://www.businessweek.com/print/magazine/content/05_13/b3926099_mz057.htm?chan=mz& on March 22, 2005.

my heart was energized with calm feelings. The interplay of these two centers was deeply enjoyable. It was an integrated, zone-like state.

The HeartMath researchers have discovered that it's surprisingly easy to prove that intuition exists, and that its accuracy increases when our feelings are deliberately harmonized. Subjects were shown random images of soothing subjects, interspersed with emotionally disturbing images. Monitoring the subjects' EEG (brain waves), ECG (electrocardiogram), and heart rate variability showed that they reacted emotionally to the images 5 to 7 seconds *before* an image appeared. Confirming the old cliché that woman are more intuitive than men, the female subjects reacted with greater accuracy and sensitivity.[20]

As we saw in the last chapter, people who practiced the HeartMath techniques were more likely to report "spiritual" experiences. ("Subjective reports from numerous individuals practiced in self-generating states of psychophysiological coherence indicate that this mode is associated with increased spiritual experience.")

In this book, I make a distinction between religious belief and spiritual practice. To my way of thinking, religion is a formal system of prayer and worship, study and conduct, aimed at pleasing God and increasing human happiness by cultivating expansive actions and attitudes such as love, kindness, generosity, etc., while spirituality includes practices

---

20 Gabriella Boehmer, "The Sixth Sense—More and More, Science Supports It," HeartMath Institute; the study referenced is: McCraty, R., Atkinson, M., Bradley, R. T., "Electrophysiological Evidence of Intuition: Part 1. The Surprising Role of the Heart," *Journal of Alternative and Complementary Medicine*, Feb 2004, Vol. 10, No. 1: 133–43; McCraty, R., Atkinson, M., Bradley, R. T., "Electrophysiological Evidence of Intuition: Part 2. A System-Wide Process?" *Journal of Alternative and Complementary Medicine*, Apr 2004, Vol. 10, No. 2: 325–36.

for directly *experiencing* God's love and guidance inwardly.

Some religious teachers would have us believe it presumptuous to try to commune with God before we die. But for those who feel a present need for a higher guidance, love, and joy, perhaps it's a worse desecration to suppress that desire.

I think the point, for athletes, is that expansive thoughts, actions, and feelings have been scientifically shown to boost fitness, health, and happiness. This much, at least, we can test in the laboratory of our bodies, hearts, and minds. And if our "quality experiences" seem to come from a higher source that's concerned for our welfare, that's all well and good. But if not, equally fine. Speaking for myself, I would rather pour my energy into *experiencing* the harmony zone, than waste time arguing about whether my experiences conform to someone's personal interpretations of scripture.

THE REST OF THE BOOK:

JOYFUL SPORTS IN THE REAL WORLD

7. THE HAPPINESS ADVANTAGE FOR RUNNERS

I spied a friend nibbling samples at the hot station in Trader Joe's. I ambled over and smiled at the Gray-Haired Guy at the oven.

"Hey, they're playing the worst songs of our generation," I quipped.

Oops. Gray Hair wasn't amused. Frowning, he opined, "Actually, they wrote some *great* songs in the Fifties and Sixties, and the one playing now is one of them."

Right. I don't remember which song it was.

Perhaps it was "Oh Where Can My Baby Be."

Or "Feelings."

I nodded politely and moved on.

For your edification, here are the worst songs ever written, according to *Dave Barry's Book of Bad Songs*:

"MacArthur Park," sung by Richard Harris

"Yummy Yummy Yummy (I Got Love In My Tummy)," performed by Ohio Express

"(You're) Having My Baby," by Paul Anka

"Honey," by Bobby Goldsboro

"Timothy," by The Buoys

"Achy Breaky Heart," by Billy Ray Cyrus

At my age, most rock music sounds like the Army's eighty-four-ton Ground Combat Vehicle driving through a liquor store.

Nevertheless, science has decided that rock music is good for us, according to a report on the *Brain Mysteries* website: *"Pump up the music—especially the bass—to make you feel powerful."*

No doubt the article will help you get pumped for football. But if you're looking for something pleasant and light to read, don't bother.

As usual, the whitecoats killed the music by turning it every which way including upside-down, while laying their little rulers along the edges and weighing and smelling and probably even licking it.

"We chose to manipulate bass levels in music because existing literature suggests that bass sound and voice are associated with dominance," Hsu says. They also observed that bass sound and voice are frequently utilized in popular culture to project perceptions of dominance and confidence. (Think James Earl Jones as Darth Vader in Star Wars.*)[21]*

Bass music makes an athlete's blood boil! Gee, who knew?

But it begs the question: Is dominance what athletes really need?

The HeartMath studies cited earlier tell us that feelings of beating down others are *not* conducive to sports performance. The opposite is also true; HeartMath researchers found that our hearts are able to work more efficiently, even at high running speeds, when we harmonize their rhythms with positive feelings such as love, kindness, compassion, and joy.

When I jog through the Stanford sports complex, I'm amazed, and not a little distressed, to hear loudspeakers

---

21. "Pump up the music—especially the bass—to make you feel powerful." BrainMysteries, http://www.sciencedaily.com/releases/2014/08/140805132250.htm.

blaring negative lyrics.

I'm not saying the Stanford football team should listen to "My Favorite Things" or "What a Wonderful World."

But I'm pretty sure that head coach David Shaw would do his guys a favor if he played tunes that stimulate will power while harmonizing their hearts for optimal performance.

Shawn Achor's book *The Happiness Advantage* is a revolutionary addition to the literature on the many links between positive feelings and success.

While a grad student at Harvard, Achor served as a proctor, a role in which he had hundreds of conversations with undergrads. Over endless cups of coffee at Starbucks, he realized that the most successful students were the ones who were habitually happy.

Achor ended up teaching the most popular course at Harvard, on the principles of positive psychology. Today, he applies those principles to help business managers rescue their companies and further their careers.

Achor realized that our traditional assumptions about happiness and success are backwards.

Most people assume that they'll be happy *after* they achieve material success. But Achor found that the opposite is true—people who are happy from the get-go are far more likely to be successful in business, relationships, or sports.

These findings blend seamlessly with three streams of ideas in this book.

First, they confirm the HeartMath findings that positive, expansive feelings boost mental and physical performance.

Second, they confirm the discovery by neuroscientists that people with high levels of activity in the brain's prefrontal cortex—the part of the brain where happy attitudes, positive expectations, will power, and the ability to achieve long-term goals are localized—are uniformly more successful than those with weaker prefrontal activation.

Finally, Achor's research confirms the long-term studies—think millennia—of the meditative traditions of the East, which tell us that placing our attention gently in the prefrontal cortex, at a point behind and between the eyebrows, is a powerful aid to calming and focusing the mind and tapping a source of inner peace, intuition, and bliss. The Eastern teachings also confirm that positive feelings support health and well-being.

Finding the energy to perform well isn't a question of beating-down our competitors, or cultivating feelings of brute dominance. It's about creating a powerful, positive flow of energy, accompanied by expansive feelings that can help our hearts, bodies, and brains perform at their best.

8. BURNOUT

On a spring morning in 1972, I joined a handful of runners at Angell Field on the campus of Stanford University for a run in the hills. The group included Peter Wood, MD, a well-known researcher on fitness and heart disease at Stanford Medical School, and Joe Henderson, founding editor of *Runner's World*. I was excited to be with these running elders, and eager to listen and learn.

There was a young man in our group whose college track coach was Laszlo Tabori, a Hungarian who placed fourth in the 1500m and sixth in the 5000m at the 1956 Olympics.

Tabori was a devotee of interval training. The young runner laughed as he recalled how he would collapse on his bed after each day's hard interval session, too exhausted to even think of doing schoolwork. His best races came after he left college and began giving his body more rest.

Interval training is supported by a large body of research. It has helped countless runners tune their bodies to race well. But like any training method, it needs to be tempered with caution. And, too often, "caution" is the last word runners want to hear.

We pounce on new methods that promise rapid results. "If intervals will make me fast, and *more* intervals will make me faster—bring 'em on!"

It's logical! More is better. But, of course, how logical is it, in reality? It's logic that's divorced from the real world—it's abstract reasoning that hops blithely over contradicting evidence. It isn't calm, objective reason; it's logic gone mad, being led around on a leash by personal emotions.

The unspoken subtext is: "I *want desperately* to be fast, to be exceptional, to shine before my peers—and I'll do *anything* to get there." But reason that doesn't include a calm, mature acceptance of reality has a way of leading us into a pit.

Athletes are notorious for cloaking their unspoken desires with noble-sounding words. We don't want to be wimps. We want to be rugged. We want to work hard. We want to accomplish. We want to do our best. We want to be heroic. We want to reap the great rewards that come by daring greatly.

We're seldom eager to hear: "Intervals are good *within reason,* in the right number, at the right pace, at the appropriate time. After building a base of aerobic fitness, intervals applied wisely can bring out the last measure of our speed."

Scratching out a training plan that's based on abstract numbers is a good first step, but it should be a tentative one. Arriving at the track for a session of speedwork, our bodies may, in fact, be sending us messages that contradict our noble plans: "I need to do this workout carefully, while monitoring my intuitive sense of my body's needs. When I exceed my body's abilities, my heart feels restless, shaky, bruised, and abused. But when I harmonize my heart's feelings before I do any fast running, my calm feelings, balanced by calm reason and experience, tell me how many intervals I can safely do and how fast I should do them. I come out of those runs feeling positive, energized, and healthy."

Training is an endless quest for balance, where the pure logic of theory is continually adjusted to the reality of our daily, individual needs. Pure logic is reliable on the plane of deep abstraction. But calm, intuitive feeling tells us what we can safely get away with in the real world, with its ever-changing ebbs and flows, and its endless outside influences. Intuitive feeling doesn't replace reason; it's reason's indispensable partner.

How does intuition work? The voice that nature uses to tell us which actions will bring us health and happiness is calm, intuitive feeling, partnered with calm, dispassionate reason. If we're unable to hear the heart's messages, it may be because, in our culture, we've chosen to emphasize reason and logic too exclusively, and we've driven feeling out of the picture. We tend to dismiss feeling as imprecise and "unscientific." As a result, we fail to realize that reason is *more* reliable when it's balanced by the heart.

I'll share a passage from Laurens van der Post's fascinating book, *The Lost World of the Kalahari*. I include it because it gives the flavor of intuition as it's experienced by people whose lives are unencumbered by the Western obsession with logic. As the story begins, the author is returning with a group of Bushmen after a long day's hunt. The Bushmen have chased a pack of eland to exhaustion. Van der Post estimates that by the end of the day they've run more than 50 miles.

Riding with one of the hunters, van der Post says, "I wonder what they'll say at the sip-wells when they learn that we've killed an eland?"

"Excuse me, Master," the Bushman says, "they already know."

When van der Post asks him to clarify, he says, "We Bushman have a wire (telegraph) here," he tapped his chest, "that brings us news."

Long before the truck arrives at the Bushmen's camp, they hear singing in the darkness.

"Do you hear that, oh, my Master?" Dabe said, whistling between his teeth. "Do you hear? They're singing 'The Eland Song.'"

Whether by "wire," or by what mysterious means, they did know at the sip-wells, and were preparing to give their hunters the greatest of welcomes. By that time we ourselves were so identified in deed as well as mind with our hosts that, despite the vast differences of upbringing and culture, their exalted mood also became our own.[22]

---

22. Laurens van der Post, *The Lost World of the Kalahari* (New York: William Morrow and Company, 1958), 255–61.

9. TRAINING IN THE AGE OF ENERGY

Can anyone doubt that the world has entered an "Age of Energy"? Of the inventions we now take for granted, few existed just 100 years ago. Electricity? Air travel? Radio? In 1900 these technologies were unknown or in their infancy. Paved roads? Few existed outside of cities.

At the end of the 19th century, a respected master of yoga in Bengal, India, published a small book, *The Holy Science*, in which he explained, based on ancient tradition, that the world had arrived at the dawn of an age of energy-awareness.

Dwapara Yuga, as it's known in the ancient texts, is the second of four ascending eras, the first of which, *Kali Yuga*, *is* characterized by ignorance of all but material realities. Writing in 1894, the yogi, Sri Yukteswar Giri, said:

With the advancement of science the world was adorned with railways, telegraphic wires and things of like nature. By the help of steam engines, electric machines and other instruments fine matters were brought into play although they were (not) clearly understood. After 1899 . . . the knowledge of the aforesaid fine matters will begin to develop and in a few years more will become so very common place that it will come within the reach of people in general.[23]

---

23. Sadhusabhapati Swami Jiu Maharaj (Swami Sri Yukteswar), *The Holy Science*, (Calcutta: Atul Chandra Chowdhary, 1920).

83

"But," you ask, "What's that got to do with running?" You might as well ask, "What's it got to do with Forty-Niner football?"

A lot, as it turns out. Bear with me as I digress yet again. In fact, San Francisco Forty-Niner coach Bill Walsh's innovative style of football, which was based on efficient application of energy for the greatest possible gain with the least effort, primarily using high-percentage short passes, changed football (and sports) forever.

The "West Coast offense," which at first was derided as sissified because it didn't apply brute force to overpower an opposing team's defenses, was incredibly successful—it brought the 49ers five Super Bowl championships, three during Walsh's tenure.

West Coast football was exciting. As executed by Hall of Fame quarterbacks Joe Montana and Steve Young, it was football re-energized, freed at least to a degree from brute materialistic consciousness.

Enough already—what's that got to do with running?

Again, a great deal.

Within my lifetime, sports training has changed radically. In 1960, when I was a high school JV guard having my nose bloodied by guards and tackles who outweighed me by 100 pounds, coaches still preached a smash-mouth, head-on, fundamentalist flavor of the football religion. I vividly recall a practice where my best friend, Bruce Fassett, and I faced off and, egged-on by Coach, did an all-out, head-on tackle drill that left us both, I'm sure, with permanent brain damage, which is why you're able to read these words today.

Today's coaches are smarter. With Walsh in the lead, first coaches in the NFL, and then their brethren at the college and high-school levels, realized that it's silly to go *through* an opposing team's defenses, when you can more easily go *over* or *around them,* with less energy and greatly increased chances of success.

The 49ers soon found it difficult to retain their assistant coaches, who were wooed away by lucrative offers of head-coaching jobs. It was a mass emigration, as a steady stream of Niner assistants packed their bags for Denver, Minneapolis, Green Bay, and other points, where they taught the West Coast game to the next generation.

Meanwhile, the training of runners had greatly changed as well. In the 1940s, '50s, and '60s, old-world coaches from Germany and Hungary pushed runners through brutal interval workouts. Mihaly Igloi, Laszlo Tabori, Waldemar Gerschler, and Franz Stampfl brooked no back-chat from their athletes, expecting them to follow the day's rigid schedules to the letter, without complaint or questioning.

Then, in the 1960s, Bill Bowerman at the University of Oregon and Arthur Lydiard in New Zealand quietly nurtured a generation of runners who would blow the interval-trained athletes away.

Bowerman was initially mocked by other college coaches who laughed at his "hard/easy" system, which aimed to apply each runner's energies most efficiently, with respect for their individual talents.

Lydiard's runners, meanwhile, were considered freaks for training like marathon runners instead of track speedsters. But the mockers fell silent when the Oregon and New Zealand teams began dominating the distance events at the NCAA championships and Olympics.

The old assumption was that the body would do whatever a runner's will could impose on it: the hardest-training runner, the one who could endure the most pain, would win. It was logical! But the new way said that each body is unique; thus Bowerman gave Steve Prefontaine harder workouts than Kenny Moore, because Moore's body took longer to recover. By tuning their training to their individual abilities, Bowerman helped both runners make the most of their talents.

Running well isn't only about bashing the body with will power, as Alberto Salazar's heroic but health-destroying efforts at Boston and New York demonstrated. For years after those races, Salazar suffered from paralyzing fatigue and chronic depression.

Today's marathon champions train smarter —the Kenyans train *very* hard when it's called for and *very* easy when it isn't. Former *Runner's World* editor Joe Henderson, now in his 60s, tells how he was able to keep up easily during a recovery run with a group of elite Kenyans who were staying at the same hotel before the New York City Marathon—and how the next day the Africans ran three minutes per mile faster.

We now know that the greatest improvements come by efficiently managing our energy. As Timothy Noakes, MD, observes in *Lore of Running,* it's always best to try to get the maximum training effect from the least effort. Training that increases, preserves, and wisely applies energy is good; training that wastes, depletes, or misapplies energy is counterproductive.

Energy-based training is simple to understand and apply. When you run, check your energy. If you "listen" carefully, your body will tell you how long and hard it can safely train. When you feel energetic, your body and mind will be eager to run, but when you're overtrained or simply tired, your mind and body will want to shuffle. Overriding those signals with brute will is a sure recipe for stalled, or even backwards progress.

There are, of course, obvious physical signals. When our legs feel dead, depleted of energy; when our heart feels bruised; when our brains are dull and our emotions are jumpy and hyper-reactive—these are clear signs that it's time to give the body a rest.

Training is simple: do lots of medium-paced aerobic running to build endurance, and do a little sub-anaerobic threshold tempo running. Fill in with very easy running to build a big base. Then follow the base months with speedwork leading up to a key race.

It absolutely requires energy to build a better body. So never train hard when your energy is low. You'll just be stealing energy from the runs that count.

Of course, the science of energy has many dimensions—diet, sleep, distance, frequency, speed—all of which demand careful attention.

In the 1970s, I would often drive to San Francisco on a Saturday morning for a long run. Afterward, I would walk around with my camera, taking pictures and thinking deep thoughts.

One day, I chanced upon a city park where a tag football game was in progress. But it was no ordinary game. It was the San Francisco city flag football league championship, and it was a heck of a contest. A spectator told me that many of the players had NFL-level talent but were too small to play with the pros. They were incredibly good, blazingly fast and agile. What I remember about the game is my impression of the tremendous energy the players were expending.

Years later, in the late 1980s, we lived in the foothills of the Sierra Nevada near Nevada City, California. We had terrible TV reception, and I rigged an amplified RV antenna so we could watch the 49ers and Hall of Fame quarterback

Joe Montana. On Sunday afternoons my wife and I would don our 49er hats, make a big bowl of popcorn, and settle in for three hours of stunningly good football.

I enjoyed those games very much—it was irresistible to watch the game played with such amazing intelligence and energy. Yet I couldn't help feeling that professional football was a deeply flawed game, albeit one played brilliantly.

I hadn't forgotten that San Francisco flag championship game, which had a faster, more upbeat, True Sport flavor than the Neanderthal, bog-snorkeling, bash-me-injure-me aspects of the pro game.

Even the airy-fairy 49er West Coast offense couldn't escape the brutal nature of the game. Quarterbacks, more than ever, were targeted and sometimes deliberately injured. And many of those short, highly efficient passing routes ended in a violent collision with a linebacker or safety.

What will happen to running, as our sport becomes increasingly energy-aware? I believe we're several steps ahead of football, which, after all, is a sport whose soul lives in the paintings of Pieter Brueghel.

The materialistic age was about rigid rules and institutional authority. In sports, athletes trained by inflexible systems and were expected to vow unconditional obedience to an authoritarian coach.

In the age of energy, it will be recognized that institutions exist to serve the needs of the individual, and that each of us has unique needs. The "system" will be based on *whatever expands the individual's awareness and gives him or her greater joy*. Sports training, too, will focus on the needs of the individual. More and more, the "coach" will be our own body, and the "textbook" will be the higher, intuitive wisdom of the heart.

10. TRAINING IN THE AGE OF ENERGY— PART 2

When I started writing *The Joyful Athlete*, I considered alternate titles: *Runner's Intuition, Heart of a Runner, Happy Heart Training*. In the end, I decided *The Joyful Athlete* was best.

I chose a title that didn't have "running" in it because I didn't want to limit the insights I'd gained to a single sport.

The *patterns* of training are the same. They're universal. Whether we run, lift weights, swim, or play basketball, tennis, football, or soccer, training is about nudging the body to do more, then letting it rest and get stronger. Only the details differ.

This was made clear to me several years ago when I picked up a book by Clarence Bass. Now in his 70s, Clarence is a former world-champion bodybuilder.

His sport is *sooooooo* different from mine. What could he possibly say that would help my running?

A lot, as it turned out.

When Clarence wrote *Challenge Yourself*, he was over 60 and had lifted weights for 50 years. In the process, he'd refined his awareness of what counted and what he could safely set aside. When I adapted his ideas, I found that they applied beautifully.

In *The Lost World of the Kalahari*, quoted earlier, Laurens van der Post tells about a South African man he met who inherited a farm but knew absolutely nothing about farming. He plunged into a study of agriculture, reading books, talking with farmers, and writing to experts, and in the end he was very successful. Along the way, he discovered that by studying one subject in great depth, he had developed an uncanny ability to learn other fields with ease.

When we become very good at one thing, we develop an energy and awareness that helps us excel elsewhere. Vaslav Nijinsky, the famous Russian ballet dancer (1889–1950), was vacationing at a Swiss ski resort, where he watched a professional skier demonstrate some fancy moves. Nijinsky donned skis and repeated the moves exactly, although he'd never skied.

What patterns of training did Clarence Bass identify that can help a runner? Here's an obvious one: recovery is crucial. No big revelation! But Bass carefully refined his understanding of recovery. At age 60-plus, he found that by training *very* easily on his off-days, and taking *many* easy days, he could train *very* hard in his main workouts, and make faster progress than at any other time in his career. Not surprisingly, the elite Africans also train "very hard/very easy."

When I adapted similar principles in my running, I got encouraging results. Instead of focusing on mileage—a questionable endeavor at age 70-plus—I put most of my energy into the weekly long run. During most of those runs, which were 2 to 3 hours, I did some speedwork—usually a 25-minute effort at above 90% of maximum heart rate. Or I would do some all-out 2-minute repeats. During the week, I ran easily and did some walking.

However, I soon discovered that it worked better to skip the hard stuff on long runs, because I recovered faster.

Combining long runs and speedwork was an inefficient way to manage my energy.

Mind you, at my age, the details of my training are *not* relevant for younger or more talented athletes. My body needs *much* more rest than it did 40 years ago. But the *principles* of energy-management are the same.

It's really a question of scale. As I mentioned, the world-leading Africans run *very* easy on their recovery days. The difference is that their "easy" runs are as fast as my medium-paced runs, and their hard efforts come 6 hours after an easy jog, instead of up to 7 days later, as mine do.

The patterns of energy-management are equal, but with the Kenyans the energy flow is vastly expanded. The details are different, but the *principles* are the same.

Clarence Bass also found that the body loves variety. Again, no surprise. Changing our training helps us stay motivated and stimulates the body to improve.

Which is my long-winded way of warming up to write, once again, about Bill Walsh, and how he applied creative energy-management principles to transform the San Francisco 49ers.

Walsh took the Niners to three Super Bowl championships, after inheriting a 2-14 team that, in the words of 49er offensive lineman Randy Cross, was "the worst 2-14 team in the history of the NFL." Yet Walsh's first Super Bowl victory came just three years after he arrived. Walsh transformed the team by applying energy-management principles that are equally applicable to running, business, relationships—anything we do.

I recently reread Walsh's classic book, *Building a Champion: On Football and the Making of the 49ers*, coauthored with journalist Glenn Dickey. What inspired me to pick it up was a run in San Francisco.

As usual, I started at Crissy Field and ambled across the Golden Gate Bridge, then onto the trails of the Marin Headlands. It's a lovely route that refreshes my spirits after a week sitting in front of the computer.

On the return, I came off the bridge and pushed the pace. I was flying along a sidewalk by the Bay, when I heard a familiar voice. I glanced ahead and saw a former 49er player from the team's glory years. I won't mention his name, except to say that he's a Hall of Fame safety, the best ever to play the game, that his initials are R. L., and that he wore number 42.

Seeing Ronnie—uh, the player—reminded me of those Sunday afternoons in the eighties when my ex-wife and I would make popcorn, don our 49ers hats, and settle in to watch Montana, Rice, and R. L. dismantle teams that practiced a traditional, grind-'em-out style of football.

What made those games enthralling was that they were about *energy*.

Bill Walsh was the Energy Master. Walsh rebuilt the 49er organization from the ground up, and the new structure was based entirely on using energy wisely. Whether he was promoting upbeat attitudes of service among the people who answered the phones and sold tickets, or designing pass plays for Montana and Rice, he was obsessed with enabling a powerful, uninterrupted energy-flow, toward the goal of winning the Super Bowl.

Walsh was quick to rid the 49ers of people and systems that created blocks in that positive energy. On the playing field, his system, which New York Giants coach Bill Parcells sneeringly dubbed the "West Coast offense," consisted of an energy-efficient style of play that Walsh had learned, in part, from head coaches Paul Brown of the Cincinnati Bengals and

Sid Gilman of the San Diego Chargers.

Brown, Gilman, and Walsh realized that the most efficient way to move the ball, with the least effort and highest odds of success, was the short pass. When applied against teams that relied on brute power, Walsh's energy-efficient plays were devastating. His system spread like wildfire, as teams lured the Niners assistants away with lucrative job offers.

I don't think it's an exaggeration to say that Walsh helped reinvent sports, and that it was important that he do so.

I mentioned in the last chapter an ancient prediction that the world has now entered an age of energy-awareness. In the last 200 years, the new energy-consciousness has flooded our lives with monster machines and tiny gadgets fueled by energy derived from coal, gas, and electricity. On a human scale, more flowing, flexible, energy-based patterns are emerging in all areas of our lives, including business, religion, and sports.

By demonstrating that intelligent use of energy is the key to success even in a Neanderthal sport like pro football, Bill Walsh served as a standard bearer for the energy age.

A simple example. When Walsh arrived in San Francisco, he was forced to fire many substandard players who had no hope of ever succeeding in the NFL. Many of the remaining players were well below NFL standards, yet Walsh treated them with respect. He poured energy into helping them improve their skills, such as they were. It was an expression of his belief that creating a powerful flow of energy in a positive *direction* is what counts.

It was a striking expression of a principle that J. Donald Walters calls "directional relativity." In his wonderful book, *Out of the Labyrinth: For Those Who Want to Believe, But Can't*, Walters argues that values are relative, but *directional*. Thus, actions that would be positive and expansive for one person (a lazy slob takes a job at a car wash) would be contractive for someone whose awareness is more expanded (Mother Teresa switches careers to wash cars).

The actions that have the highest value for humanity are those that expand happiness and decrease suffering. An immutable law of nature says that expansive actions always give us an inflow of joy.

A simple example from running, mentioned in the last chapter. When Kenny Moore ran at Oregon, coach Bill Bowerman assigned him a "hard/easy" schedule of workouts, recognizing that Moore needed more rest than Steve Prefontaine. Both runners were intent on improving—moving forward in an expansive direction—but Moore needed to take a slightly different route to the same goal; he needed easier training than "Pre."

If values were fixed and inflexible, Moore and Prefontaine would have thrived on the same training. If values were anchored in stone, all runners could read the same book and follow its schedules to the letter. But it's obvious that the *individual* needs to adapt his or her training in ways that expand his/her own fitness, not someone else's.

Walsh understood that creating powerful, positive energy required working sensitively with the individual player. He knew that helping each 49er player improve, even the worst, was the key to building a successful organization.

In Walsh's words:

> We set about teaching fundamentals and skills, establishing a system of football on offense and defense, and establishing a positive atmosphere and attitude.

> We were enthusiastically involved in developing the players we had, trying to improve their consistency and effectiveness. I think our staff did an admirable job the

first two years, working in most cases with men who could not compete in the NFL, developing them to their fullest potential. (*Building a Champion*, p. 93)

Sports is changing. Walsh was among the first coaches in pro football to devote so much energy to developing the individual player, even the least-talented, as a key to the team's success. He wanted positive energy to permeate the organization, with no small pockets of poisonous discontent.

When superstar quarterback Joe Montana joined the Niners, Walsh didn't immediately insert him in games, in hopes of improving the team's woeful record. Instead, he spent many months helping him refine his basic quarterbacking skills, such as his footwork, and only used Montana in plays where he stood a good chance of experiencing success and gaining confidence.

Energy was the key. By helping the individual optimize his energy, he developed a team of players who were faster, smarter, more energy-efficient and positive than any other. The "system" proved itself with five Super Bowl wins, three in Walsh's time.

What can runners learn from Clarence Bass and Bill Walsh about managing energy? I suspect it's the notion of studying our "energy economy" and adopting the methods that work best for us, at our level.

No two runners are alike. How quickly do *our* bodies recover? Reviewing our training diary, we can identify the most effective interval between our long and hard runs.

Which runs leave us feeling energized—"pleasantly tired," as Arthur Lydiard suggested—rather than overextended and sandbagged? Where are the personal "edges" we can nudge to become faster, stronger, more enduring and energized? How far can we press our edges without overtraining? How much rest do *we* need, compared to other runners? What heart rates leave us feeling best during daily runs? Long runs? Speedwork? Races? How often do we need a brutal, breakout run to prompt our body to rise to the next level?

The way we feel while running can help us find the answers. When we cooperate with nature, it rewards us with positive feelings. The best runs feel "expansive."

It's difficult for most runners to stay always inside nature's fences—never straying beyond their present capabilities, never pretending they're better than they are. Yet progress begins with truthfully admitting where we stand.

Once we know what our bodies are capable of, we can train expansively and rise to the next rung.

We can choose a diet that gives us energy. We all need carbs and protein, but the specifics are individual. My roommate and I eat radically different foods. About the only food we can share is pizza. But we both eat the same "food groups."

We can cultivate positive feelings, which dramatically increase the power output of the heart. We can get enough sleep. And, like Bill Walsh, we can eliminate "energy killers" from our lives—negative people, junk food, overtraining, etc. We can sing, whistle, smile, and help others. We can train in places where we feel good.

The energy we get from positive people, music, books, movies, art, and scenery is an "ergonomic aid," because it lifts our mood and boosts our immune system, which is vitally involved in recovery.

We can plan our training for the months and years ahead, but adjust it daily. The body's needs change continually, and calm, objective feeling can help us know if we're doing the right training, moment by moment. There's an upbeat feeling when we're on the right track. Good energy feels good.

Postscript: I was delighted to receive a note from Clarence Bass after I posted this chapter online. I don't know how Clarence found it, but I'm touched and impressed by his expansive spirit. At 70-plus, he may no longer move the weights he did at 40. But he continues to move and inspire others.

11. NATURAL ZONES

Are there natural training "zones" in running?

I think so. At least, my body tells me there are paces it likes best.

During the warmup, for example, my body seems to "want" to run no faster than about 65% to 67% of maximum heart rate.

Researchers have found that at 65% of MHR, the heart does an interesting thing. As I mentioned in chapter 5, a measurement called "heart rate variability" (HRV) suddenly gets faster.

It's a bit of a mental stretch to understand HRV. Simply put, our heart rate changes continually, and HRV is a measure of how often the heart changes speeds in a given time.

As we saw in chapter 5, researchers at Heartmath Institute discovered that HRV reflects our positive or negative feelings. Happy, expansive feelings make the heart change speeds smoothly—the HRV curve looks smooth and harmonious (figure 1, chapter 5). But negative feelings such as anger and fear make the heart shift gears erratically and inefficiently—the HRV curve looks jagged and irregular.

When the HRV curve is smooth and regular, the heart can work more efficiently, and its electrical power output increases by up to 380%. For optimal running, it's important to tune the heart so it can change speeds smoothly.

Years ago, I ran with a friend who always warmed up slowly. I hadn't yet discovered the magic of the long warmup, and the slow pace drove me nuts. Yet those runs always ended well. As we picked up the pace, I was able to sail along much more comfortably than on solo runs, after my usual brief or nonexistent warmup.

At 65% MHR, the heart suddenly starts to change speeds much more rapidly. My theory—that's all it is, I have no data for this—is that 65% is approximately the top speed at which the body "wants" to warm up. My only evidence is that it feels right—my runs go better when I stay under 65% to 67% until going faster feels easy.

I wouldn't blame you for dismissing these ideas as candidates for the Annals of Kooky Sports Science—if it weren't for the fact that I *always* have better runs when I warm up at the sub-65% pace. And I'm not terribly ashamed that I can't back up these ideas with research. As we know from the successful training methods of Arthur Lydiard, empirical evidence—our own direct experience—is a valid foundation for a training plan; in fact, the lore of empirically based training is miles ahead of sports science.

I suspect the reason my body and heart don't feel right when I run faster during the warmup is because there's important work that the body must do before it can go faster with ease, and it's done best below the 65% warmup threshold. It seems reasonable, for example, that the heart would "want" to find a smooth, efficient rhythm before it starts changing speeds more rapidly.

For these reasons, I suspect that "under 65%" is a natural training zone. Are there others?

In *Heart Monitor Training for the Compleat Idiot*, John L. Parker Jr. advises us to do most runs no faster than 70% of

MHR, calculated by the Karvonen formula (maximum heart rate minus resting heart rate, times 0.7, plus resting heart rate).

When I asked Parker how he arrived at the 70% figure, his answer was vague. I wasn't satisfied—I wanted hard numbers; I wanted to know the precise, *best* way to train. But after several years of experimenting with the 70% Karvonen heart rate, I did an about-face. I now believe that Parker was thoroughly justified in saying "This is the way it is. Just do it."

In the early 1970s, Parker trained with Olympians Frank Shorter, Jeff Galloway, and Jack Bacheler. I suspect that, like most elites, he evolved his methods by monitoring the feedback from his own body. His unshakable confidence in the 70% figure was born of his experience while training for years at an elite level, as well as the successes of the thousands of runners who followed his system.

Lab studies begin to take a backseat, when we've had the experience of running in the "harmony zone," where our body tells us, unmistakably: "This is the right way to train."

Those feelings, in my experience, come at distinct heart rates during different phases of a run. During the warmup, they come at about 65% to 67% MHR.

During a transition phase to a faster, "aerobic-metabolism-improvement" pace, the feeling of *rightness* seems to come at around 70% to 75% of MHR.

Finally, during the aerobic-improvement phase, those feelings of rightness are strongest at about 70% of MHR per the Karvonen formula—as Parker predicted.

For me, 70% Karvonen translates as about 78-79% of maximum heart rate, calculated as a straight percentage. In fact, during long runs, if I'm rested, fit, and thoroughly warmed up, it feels wonderful to lock into the 70% Karvonen pace. But if I let my pace wander above 80%, the feeling changes. I don't even need to check the heart monitor—I'll feel a slight disharmony, and when I glance at the monitor, sure enough, I'll see that I've drifted above 80%. When I slow and my heart rate falls back under 80%, I feel fine again. But if I persist in running faster than 80%, I'm unable to run as far, and it feels like a "slow race," as if I'm borrowing resources from the next run.

Are 65% and 80% (or 70% Karvonen) two of the body's natural "training zones"?

I suspect the answer, as so often happens, is "yes and no."

Yes, because there's surely an optimal, individual warmup pace, which may hover just under 65%.

And it stands to reason that, for each runner, there's a personal optimal aerobic improvement pace, and an optimal speedwork pace for improving anaerobic function, and then a best speedwork pace for improving leg speed.

A chart on page 282 of Tim Noakes's *Lore of Running* (4th ed.) shows five training "zones" defined by Sally Edwards and Edmund Burke. The chart shows how the zones get slower as we age and our max heart rate decreases.

I mention the chart because it's more evidence that we shouldn't let fixed numbers be our guide. First, because the optimal training zones change with age; and second, because they vary individually at any age. And they vary with countless other factors, such as fatigue, illness, weather, etc.

The *principle* of zones is valid, but hard numbers should be taken as starting points for individual experimentation.

An interesting feature of the Edwards/Burke chart is that it shows how the heart zones "slip" as we grow older. That is, the optimal aerobic improvement pace not only gets lower as we advance in years, but it occurs at a lower percentage of maximum heart rate. When I was 30, I suspect my optimal aerobic improvement pace was closer to 85% MHR, while at age 71 it's just under 80%.

Arthur Lydiard recommended that aerobic improvement runs be done at "medium" pace, by which he meant a high aerobic pace. In his excellent book on Lydiard's training methods, *Healthy Intelligent Training*, Keith Livingstone places that optimal aerobic pace at about 85% of MHR, but it's clear that he's talking about younger runners.

Which zone-based training system is best? John L. Parker's? Philip Maffetone's? Arthur Lydiard's?

Some runners prefer to do year-round aerobic training, with regular speedwork thrown in, Frank Shorter being an elite example. Others prefer periodized training, toward the goal of peaking for an important race.

In either system, the *proportion* of hard and easy running is a key factor. Lydiard believed that running tons of miles at a high aerobic pace prepares the body for faster training and racing. He felt that doing any anaerobic running during the base-building period decreases the aerobic training effect.

Lydiard's training was beautiful, in the sense that it was wonderfully balanced. More than any other coach, he was attuned to the body's need for variety, from very slow jogging on recovery days, to fast aerobic running to develop endurance-at-speed, to hill work for strength and form; long intervals for anaerobic endurance, and short speedwork for leg speed.

Of these variations, he felt that the great pool of aerobic work was, by far, the most important. It was the base from which all other training draws energy. A runner had to return to the aerobic "source" again and again to renew and build his strength.

I recently watched a DVD of legendary cellist Mstislav Rostropovich playing the Bach Cello Suites. It was amazingly wonderful. I arrived home exhausted and turned it on and lay on the bed and let the music wash over me. My brain was too fried to analyze the music, so I simply drank it in with my cells. I felt that Bach's music was tapping the joy of a higher, spiritual world and filling the room with blessings.

In his introductory remarks, Rostropovich explains that Bach allows the musical line (in the Suites, there are often no melodies) to drop low, in order, as he puts it, "to gather energy." Then, Bach ascends and explores ethereal realms until the energy runs out and he has to descend and collect energy again.

Training is like that: it's about proportion, balance, and moderation. Like Bach's music, honoring its wonderful precision opens doors to enjoyment and success.

12. HOW TO INCREASE YOUR MILEAGE ENJOYABLY

It seems entirely reasonable: surely, the best way to increase mileage is to run everything slowly. The running will be easy, we won't risk overtraining, and we'll be able to rack up the miles.

Strange to say, even though it sounds logical, it's wrong.

At least, that's my experience. I spent 15 years training slowly for ultramarathons. During that time, 10-minute pace was typical and 9 minutes was fast.

I occasionally wondered if increasing my mileage would improve my race times; yet the thought of running more hours at a slogging pace was nauseating.

Here's the funny thing. The moment I began training *faster*, my enthusiasm soared and I found it easy, even exciting, to pack on the miles.

What a paradox! But I believe there's a simple explanation. Not to get too complicated, but *running with the right level of energy stimulates enthusiasm*. Conversely, the wrong energy, or too little energy, puts our enthusiasm in the pits.

Training at a dreary slog improves endurance, but not speed. Much worse, training only at a slow pace teaches the body (and mind) to deliver low-level energy. The risk is that low-burner energy becomes so deadeningly boring that we stagnate. Our body is unenthusiastic, our spirits sag, our minds drift—and, just *blah!* Let's face it, it's human to want to experience high energy, because it's enjoyable!

Of course, it's dangerous to turn up the flame too high, too often. Running even a single extra mile in a long run, or a single extra 400-meter repeat on the track, can delay our recovery and our progress.

What kind of energy generates enthusiasm *and* progress?

Ancient cultures associated energy with images of fire. It's a useful system that can give us insights for managing our training wisely.

Low energy is a smoldering fire. It produces unhealthy smoke, yields little warmth, and creates a dark mood.

We experience low energy when we're ill or overtrained. When our inner fire burns low, it's hard to think about running. We sleep late, stagger out of bed, and feel irritable, sullen, defensive, resentful, reactive, and contractive. Low energy and enthusiasm aren't best friends.

The second image of energy is a fire that's raging out of control. Most runners will have little trouble recognizing this kind of energy—because we're routinely tempted to set our training ablaze. It's this raging forest fire kind of energy that most often gets us in trouble.

Let's give it an appropriate name. We'll call it "ego-active energy."[24] It's very active, which is why we love it. "Sure! I can do 12x400m in 70 seconds with a 2-minute recovery!" That's "active" energy talking. And, too often, it's *ego*-active—we push hard not because it will improve our fitness, but because we'll look good, feel proud, stand out, and get a rush.

Ego-active energy is a very, very good thing, up to a point. The problems start when we let the exciting quality of fiery

---

24. I've borrowed the term "ego-active" from J. Donald Walters' excellent book, *Education for Life*.

energy tempt us into running our bodies into a ditch.

Little wonder that a synonym for overtraining is "burnout." When we run too much, we use the fire of will to burn up the body's resources—including the healthy reserve of adaptation energy that the body needs to recover and get stronger.

Fortunately, there's a third kind of energy that, as Goldilocks said, is "just right"—it generates enthusiasm, improves fitness, and leave us feeling wonderful.

In the ancient traditions, the third level of energy was symbolized by a fire that's controlled and useful. It warms but doesn't burn. Think of a campfire on a cool fall evening, or a fire in a barbecue, cooking a delicious meal. Or a fire in the hearth on a snowy winter morning.

Do these images evoke a certain kind of running? A controlled, level-headed, moderate, effective, hard-working, intelligent, wise kind of running? A kind of training that we associate with highly successful, level-headed runners like Bob Kennedy and Frank Shorter?

That's the kind of energy we should obviously look for, if we want to improve and enjoy our training.

History's most successful distance running coach, Arthur Lydiard, encapsulated that energy in two simple words. He encouraged his athletes to finish every run feeling "pleasantly tired." That says it all.

From the time he began expounding his ideas, in the 1950s and early 1960s, Lydiard's system has produced an endless stream of Olympic medalists and world-record holders. And the essence of what he preached was *balance.*

Lydiard believed that progress requires hard work, balanced by a wise respect for the body's ever-changing needs.

Respected running journalist Rich Englehart graciously

lent me a tape of a conversation he had with Arthur Lydiard's most famous disciple, Peter Snell, winner of gold in the 800 meters at the 1960 and 1964 Olympics and the 1500 in 1964. Later, Rich wrote in an exchange of emails:

I'm a huge Lydiard fan and would agree with all the tributes he's been given for his contributions to our knowledge of training. But I think his biggest contribution by far was creating an approach that is basically enjoyable, certainly more so than the approaches I started with. I think he understood that, too.

I spend a lot of time looking at the LetsRun online forum and see so many people who want to formularize everything and have some sort of schedule and table with precise numbers to follow. The trouble with that approach is that the athlete using it is not the same person each day.

I recall someone asking Lydiard about using your heart rate when you wake up in the morning as a measure of how recovered you are, and he said, "Well, you've got to think about who you were sleeping with."

I think a big part of the fascination people have with all the physiological stuff in the sport now is that it's an approach which is quantifiable and therefore fairly easy to analyze. Try to explain to people that the reason you knocked 9 minutes from your marathon best is that you enjoyed your training most days and what you did "felt right," and most everyone will begin trying to analyze the "real" reason what you did worked so well. It's important to understand training methodology, but it's equally important to understand the individual athlete. This is the bit about training with Lydiard's methods that you can only understand from getting to know him. His genius was partly the method he devised, but it was also about understanding his athletes and knowing how to apply the method.

In *Healthy Intelligent Training: The Proven Principles of Arthur Lydiard,* Keith Livingstone writes:

On what was to be his [Lydiard's] last talk, an American coach repeatedly asked Arthur how his athletes dealt with the pain of training. Arthur didn't seem to understand the question, whichever way it was put.

In the end he responded indignantly: "My athletes didn't have to deal with the pain! We enjoyed ourselves!"

It's a telling glimpse into Lydiard's philosophy.

What follows is a bit of a ramble through Lydiard's ideas. Bear with me. In the end, I think I'll be able to show that there are sound, practical reasons for giving highest priority to running *enjoyably*.

Lydiard spent years tinkering with his own running, with a goal of discovering the best training for distance runners. Working in the "lab" of his own body, he ran up to 300 miles per week, testing various combinations of speed and distance. The system he arrived at was surprisingly simple.

In essence, Lydiard said that a talented runner should do three long runs per week—a 10-mile run at a high aerobic pace, a 15-miler at medium-aerobic pace, and a 22-miler on the weekend, after gradually working up to those distances. They can then fill in with easy running to build up to 100 miles per week. Runners with competitive goals should include two or three speedwork sessions per week in the weeks approaching a key race.

For runners shooting for peak fitness for a specific race, Lydiard recommended "periodizing" their training in four phases: aerobic conditioning, hill training for strength and flexibility, long speedwork for anaerobic conditioning, and short speedwork for leg speed.

The core of the program is the three long runs during the base-building period, and the most important of these is the weekend 22-miler. It's crucial to note that Lydiard believed the long runs should be done at "medium" or "moderate" speed—a high aerobic pace. He by no means recommended that they be done slowly, at a jogging pace, or that they include walking breaks.

Peter Snell, now a professor of cardiology and an exercise researcher at the University of Texas Southwest Medical Center in Dallas, says the reason for doing long runs at medium pace is that it exhausts the glycogen in the type IIa fast-twitch muscle fibers, forcing the trainable type IIb fast-twitch fibers to take over part of the load. Because the type IIb fibers are improvable (type IIa fibers are not), they get stimulated to produce more of their kind, and we get faster.

To exhaust the glycogen in the muscle fibers, Lydiard believed the long run should be done without taking fuels. It should be noted, however, that his runners absolutely gorged on carbs after these runs, storing adequate fuel for the next run.

Snell says that slow jogging doesn't affect the type IIb fibers the same way, and this is why people who jog through their long runs develop the ability to finish a marathon, but don't get faster.

These are plausible explanations for why Lydiard's training, based on the three long runs, improves endurance *and* speed. An equally important reason is that running at medium pace is *enjoyable*. And without enjoyment, few runners would be motivated to increase their mileage, much less build up to 100-mile weeks.

In fact, two factors make "medium-paced" running

enjoyable.

The first is the reason most exercise is enjoyable: because it generates energy. Up to a point, the more energy we channel through our physical, mental, and emotional "systems," the greater the enjoyment. Of course, if we turn up the flame too high, too often, the body gets overstressed and enjoyment evaporates.

Good training is about finding a balance where the effort is like the beneficial fire in a barbecue—not too hot, just right.

How can we balance pace, distance, and frequency and find the "just-enough" point where fitness and enjoyment expand in an optimal, healthy way?

It turns out to be surprisingly easy, because the body is happy to tell us. When we run at exactly the pace that optimally expands aerobic fitness (given all variations of weather, diet, sleep, fitness, etc.), we feel wonderful. That's the body's way of saying: "You're doing it right!"

Feelings of enthusiasm are an amazingly accurate gauge for the pace our body can safely and optimally handle for a given distance, on a given day. But we need to check our hearts for the right kind of enthusiasm—it's not the adolescent, emotional kind of excitement that always seems to lead us to do too much, but a calm, mature, controlled positive feeling.

The second factor that makes Lydiard's training enjoyable is that when we do it correctly, we don't overtrain. As I mentioned earlier, Lydiard urged his runners to finish every run feeling "pleasantly tired." And he meant it. It was a cornerstone of his system. He believed that it's important to leave some energy in the tank at the end of a run, because the body will use that "adaptation energy" to recover and improve.

What's the best way to increase your mileage safely and enjoyably? The answer is simple: by *training as enjoyably as possible.*

Lydiard gave us the formula for enjoyment: do all "aerobic improvement" runs at a medium to high aerobic pace, and always run a bit less than you could. On the "off" days, do nothing but easy running to aid recovery.

An important question remains: how can we pinpoint our own most enjoyable pace? We'll look for the answer in the next chapters.

13. *ARF! ARF!* TRAIN LIKE A DOG

When it comes to exercise, dogs are smarter than we are.

A dog will express its enthusiasm without prejudice, reservations, or a whole lot of discrimination.

You seldom have to beg a dog to chase a ball. *Yes! Yes! Let's go! Throw the ball! Now!*

For a dog, exercise isn't a burden, it's a challenge almost too exciting to bear. *We're running* 10 *miles today! Okay! Oh boy! Let's start now! Why are you sitting on the stairs?! Let's go!*

Dogs don't waste time brooding over their mistakes. *Hey! Wow! I didn't catch the ball! Great! Throw it again! Throw it again!*

Dogs don't run for health or weight-loss or longevity. They run because, well, they love to run.

And when they don't feel like running, they stop, wander under the porch, sniff the ground, turn in a circle three times, and lie down and snooze.

I've started my Bow-Wow Training Plan. As my role models, I'm choosing two runners who "train like dogs," in the body-wiggling, tongue-hanging, tail-wagging, skipping and jumping sense.

In the 1970s, 2:14 marathoner Gary Fanelli achieved notoriety for showing up at races dressed in full Blues Brothers regalia, complete with porkpie hat, white shirt, dark jacket, black tie, and shades—and then pushing the pace in the lead pack. A photo in *Runner's World* immortalized Gary's "Joliet Jake" Blues persona.

When psychologists studying elite runners tested Gary, he posted the highest scores they'd ever seen for positive attitude.

Gary still runs top times in his age group—last I heard, he'd clocked close to 50 minutes for 10 miles, at just under age 50. And he's retained his offbeat sense of humor. A recent Christmas card from Gary shows him reclining on the fender of a clapped-out car, puffing a big cigar amid his scrap metal collection.

No one personifies the joy of running more than my second role model, Joe Henderson.

Joe edited *Runner's World* from 1970, four years after the magazine was founded, until 1985, when it was purchased by Rodale and moved to Pennsylvania. Joe stayed on as a columnist until 2003, when he was let go by the magazine's increasingly marketing-driven publishers, who were intent on shifting its target demographic from Joe and Jane Runner to Brock and Tiffany Spandex. Too bad. For the magazine's best 33 years, Joe was its soul.

Joe never met a runner he didn't like. Through his *Marathon & Beyond* columns and his books, he continues to express the thoughts of Every Runner.

Several years ago, Joe and I ran 10 miles of a marathon together. If you get a chance to run with Joe, don't miss it. On the roads, in t-shirt and shorts, Joe exudes joy. If he had a tail, he'd be barred from races—the wagging would endanger the other runners.

When I started running 47 years ago at age 26, every run was an adventure. It was a chance to explore new thoughts, feelings, textures, sounds, smells, and places. I ran with the same joy on sand, pavement, grass, artificial tracks, and trails.

I trained to the music of my own heart. But when I accepted a job at *Runner's World*, I was introduced to the scientific approach, and the music stopped.

It took me 20 years to realize that science raises more questions for runners than it answers. Science studies small parts of training; it rarely looks at the whole picture.

I solved the training puzzle to my satisfaction when I discovered that my body was telling me everything I needed to achieve fitness and enjoyment together.

And, guess what? Good training turned out to be not so different from the tail-wagging, intuitive approach that got me started.

I spent two decades testing dozens of training methods. Most were dead ends. Today, four decades after I began running, I've come full circle. I'm following my Bow-Wow Training Plan that calls for running with the gusto of a hound dog.

It's Spike here, scratching at the door. *I'm ready! Let's run!*

14. TRUE SPORT AT THE OLYMPICS

Several months after the ill-fated 1972 Olympic Games, Bil Gilbert (not a typo; one "l") wrote a thoughtful article for *Sports Illustrated*.

In "Gleanings From a Troubled Time," Bil reflected on the tragic events of that year's Games, and what they might mean for the future.[25]

In the wake of the Black September murders at Munich, Gilbert found hope in the self-renewing nature of sports.

Gilbert believed that sports exists on three levels: Big Sport, True Sport, and High Sport.

Big Sport is exploding scoreboards, scantily dressed cheerleaders, and free agency. It's about money, marketing, ego, and hype.

High Sport is sports raised to the level of art. It's the Olympics at their most inspiring—think Frank Shorter's marathon gold at the '72 Games. Shorter made it look easy. While running at sub-5-minute pace, he seemed to float over the ground.

True Sport is you and I.

Gilbert wrote:

There is first True Sport, the manifestation of man's seemingly innate urge to play. True Sport is organized for and often by participants and is essentially a private

25. "Gleanings From a Troubled Time," *Sports Illustrated*, December 25, 1972.

matter like eating or making love.

It's a moody piece, but the skies clear and the sun emerges when Gilbert tells how he and a friend, a college track coach, drove four girls from the local track club to a tiny all-comers meet in a nearby town.

Gilbert contrasts the relaxed atmosphere of the show-up-and-run event with the tension and hype of the Olympics. He notes that True Sport, at the Winchester All-Comers meet, "stands to High Sport as a craft does to an art."

Big Sport, by contrast, is "a corrupted, institutionalized version of True Sport." . . . It stands to High Sport and True Sport as a molded plastic angel does to sculpture and pottery."

Gilbert's fine article has the ring of truth. The small joy of sports is an individual matter. It's about one person growing larger. True Sport expands us. High Sport shows us our potential. That's why it moves our hearts.

I've described, in another chapter, how Bill Walsh brought the values of True Sport and High Sport to Big Sport as coach of the San Francisco Forty-Niners. He showed that the values of True Sport are the surest path to success, even in the crass Big Sports arena.

Walsh's teams were incredibly entertaining to watch, and the reasons weren't hard to discern. It was because he infused his teams with expansive values.

Football practices in the NFL had traditionally tended to be mini-games in which the players were expected to beat the crap out of their teammates.

Walsh decided that brains could build great teams and win games, better than brawn. The Niners rarely practiced in full uniform. Instead, they generally worked out in shorts and jerseys, running their intricate pass patterns endlessly. Practices were as intelligently managed and time-efficient as a Joe Montana touchdown drive.

Other teams hooted at this airy-fairy brand of football—until it became apparent that the 49ers could dominate them at will. The "West Coast offense" spread throughout the league.

From an unsigned article on Yahoo:

Even a short list of Walsh's adherents is stunning. [George] Seifert, Mike Holmgren, Dennis Green, Sam Wyche, Ray Rhodes and Bruce Coslet all became NFL head coaches after serving on Walsh's San Francisco staffs, and Tony Dungy played for him. Most of his former assistants passed on Walsh's structures and strategies to a new generation of coaches, including Mike Shanahan, Jon Gruden, Brian Billick, Andy Reid, Pete Carroll, Gary Kubiak, Steve Mariucci and Jeff Fisher.

Bill Walsh proved that efficient energy-management can work wonders. The lesson has relevance for all sports.

Smash-mouth tactics rarely work in the long haul, not even in individual sports. When we yield to the temptation to log too many brutally hard runs, driven by ego and ambition, we fail.

"He [Walsh] was a perfectionist," said Keena Turner, a linebacker with the Niners for 11 years, before becoming a coach. "When writing his script, he didn't believe that running the football was the way to get there. It had to be prettier than that—beautiful in some way."

Albert Einstein said, "The pursuit of truth and beauty is a sphere of activity in which we are permitted to remain children all our lives." Forty-Niner football *was* beautiful, and it was fun to watch. When we train with harmony and expansive values, managing energy wisely, our sport can become beautiful, too.

Former 49er coach Jim Harbaugh had a photo of Walsh taped to his computer monitor. Before joining the Niners, Harbaugh spent endless hours learning from his longtime friend and mentor.

"Bill Walsh personified what it meant to be a human being," Harbaugh said. "Everything that came out of his mind, his heart, his mouth, I hung on every single word."

Even the 49er players who had smash-mouth roles— fullback Tom Rathman, center and guard Randy Cross, safety Ronnie Lott—were upbeat when reflecting on what it was like to play for Walsh.

Walsh made the 49ers a True Sport act on the Big Sport stage.

Thank you, Bill Walsh, for reminding us what matters.

15. MENTAL FOCUS OF HAPPY RUNNERS

Matt Killingsworth did his doctoral research at Harvard. For his thesis, he developed an iPhone app that allowed people to record the times of the day when they felt most and least happy.

Matt's study concluded that people are happiest when they're focusing their attention wholly in the present moment.

His findings are important for athletes.

In the early 1970s, Bruce Ogilvie and Thomas Tutko studied the mental attitudes of runners. They identified two distinct patterns, which they called "associating" and "dissociating."

The associaters kept their minds focused while they ran, deeply attentive to what they were doing, carefully monitoring their pace, breathing, posture, form, fluid intake, fuels, fatigue, etc. When their attention strayed, they patiently brought it back to the moment.

The other group, the dissociaters, let their minds drift. They believed that allowing their attention to wander led to creative insights and inspirations.

There's nothing wrong with the second style. But the first group were far more successful at achieving their competitive goals.

Killingsworth's research would seem to predict that the associaters would be not only more successful, but happier.

What does it mean to "focus"? Does focus equate to running with a jaw-grinding, tense, micromanaging state of mind?

Not at all. It's well known, in meditative spiritual circles, that mental strain destroys concentration. Trying to corral our thoughts with hard-nosed willpower simply doesn't work. Under the pressure of an overbearing will, our thoughts scatter.

Yogis, Buddhist monks, and Christian contemplatives— the practical scientists of the mind—teach that if we want to focus our attention, the most important thing is to harmonize the feelings of our heart.

A well-known spiritual teacher from the yoga tradition, Swami Kriyananda, put it like this:

> In teaching meditation, people speak of the need to calm the mind. In fact, it is the heart that needs to be calmed. That is why devotion is fundamental to success in meditation. When the heart is calm and one-pointed in its focus on God, the mind is also still, because there are no restless feelings to disturb it.

The mind-calming power of harmonious feelings is confirmed by the research of scientists at Heartmath Institute, which I summarized in chapters 5 and 6.

Next time you run, try a simple experiment. Try forcing your mind to concentrate. You'll quickly discover that it's no good. Now try dwelling *pleasantly* on each moment, on *this* moment, then the next.

As you round each bend, relax into *that* moment. Enjoy *this* scenery. Enjoy running in this new place and state.

With calm detachment, watch your body run, as if you were going along for the ride. You won't have to work hard to focus your attention, if you can achieve happy *feelings*.

The spiritual teachers tell us that concentration is synonymous with intense *interest*. It isn't about whanging the rebellious mind with a two-by-four. It's an art of balancing effort and ease in an increasingly smooth, alert flow.

Frank Shorter described elite racing as a series of surges, as the runner presses on the gas, then relaxes, takes stock, and enjoys.

It's similar with learning to focus attention. It helps to employ "surges," focusing intently on what's going on, then letting our mind and heart relax and enjoy.

After dedicating an entire run to this practice, you'll nearly always feel wonderful, even if you don't achieve perfect focus.

Just as we warm up the body before we start to run fast, the mind needs to be warmed up, too.

A friend of mine is an accomplished singer. Every year, she attends a workshop given by an internationally renowned performing group, Chanticleer.

Karen told me a surprising thing. She said the Chanticleer singers spend *one or two hours* warming up their voices before they practice or perform. During the warmup, they sing only in the low register, and they sing softly for a long time.

I think that's wonderful. As a singer, I find that it takes me 40 minutes to an hour of quiet humming and low-register singing to prepare my voice to sing loudly with effortless ease.

The Chanticleer singers told Karen that warming up in the low range reduces the risk of damaging the vocal chords, which are surprisingly fragile. It also prepares the voice to sing high. "Take care of the low register, and you won't have to worry about the high register."

In my running, I find that a long warmup pays similar dividends. I'm not sure why, but I find that it's always easier to go fast after a relaxed, gradual warmup.

It pays off mentally and emotionally as well. Gradually refining a mental focus while letting the body warm up at its own pace yields happier, more productive runs.

Tom Taylor is a friend who formerly managed a small health food store. At first, Tom *hated* to stock the shelves, feeling that it was a boring, time-consuming task that kept him from more important work.

One day, he decided to make a game of it. He put all of his attention into restocking the shelves—carefully lining up the cans and bottles, making sure that the labels faced forward, and cleaning any dust or stains from the products and shelves.

Tom quickly noticed that stocking had become a very enjoyable part of his day; soon, he was looking forward to it. Tom said that narrowly focusing his attention made him *more* aware, not less:

What I do now is not only stock shelves, but I'm aware of everything that's going on in the store while I'm doing it. I try to be aware of the customers. If I hear somebody ask for something, I tune in and get involved, and if somebody comes in, I'm talking to them. So I've made stocking shelves more than what it is. I do the best I can with every little thing I try to do, even if it's just lining up the cans perfectly, and so I enjoy it. It isn't difficult to enjoy something if you're putting your energy into it. If you're always resisting, of course it's no fun at all. I think that's the thing you start to realize, that everything can be fun if you're really there with it, and it doesn't really matter what you're doing.

I know it sounds weird, but I've been able to finish some of my *worst, most godawful* runs feeling wonderful, by focusing my attention deeply on what was happening, even the bad parts.

Focusing attention energizes the part of the brain where positive attitudes are localized: in the prefrontal cortex (PFC) and anterior cingulate gyrus. It's a reason why yogis, Buddhists, and Christian contemplatives place so much emphasis on learning to concentrate there. The PFC is a "feel-good" part of the brain. Researchers have long known that people who are good at setting and achieving long-term goals, and who have a habitually positive attitude, have strongly activated PFCs.

But there's a dangerous phase in every run where we can easily lose our focus and happiness.

Every run begins with the body. The warmup is where the body prepares to run fast. As the body finds a groove, good feelings automatically arise. The danger comes later, when the good feelings start to fade. Without strong feelings to keep our attention, the mind can easily drift away.

At that point, it's important to take control. If we let our focus weaken, we're likely to lose the happy feelings in the last stages of the run.

When our attention starts to flag, we can bring it back by deliberate effort, disciplining it like a child that wants to wander into a busy street.

The discipline needs to be gentle but persistent. We can think of this part of the run as a rite of passage—a test of our resolve to stay in joy.

When we keep control, the last part of the run can be wonderful, with attention and feelings merging in a positive, high-energy flow.

A practice that's consistently helped me create happy runs is repeating a positive affirmation, short phrase, or a verse of a song. It should be something that has personal meaning and evokes positive feelings. Or we can dwell on a pleasant memory—a time when our heart expanded and we were rewarded with feelings of love and joy. Another good way to deepen our focus is by sending positive thoughts, prayers, and blessings to others—giving ourselves an expansive incentive to discipline our attention.

Matt Killingsworth's finding that mental focus creates happiness tells us that letting our minds wander is a mistake. Not everyone will choose to be an associater. It's the more difficult path, but there's no doubt that it pays big dividends.

16. A MERRY HEART GOES ALL THE WAY

Listen to Bob Kennedy, the first American to run a sub-13-minute 5000m. Bob spent time training with the elite Kenyans at their camp in Iten. He described his experiences in a *Runner's World* interview.[26] Kennedy describes how he set out with Kenyan elite Moses Kiptanui on a 6-mile run. After 300 meters, Kiptanui announced that he was feeling too tired and went home. Three days later, he would run a world-class 7:58 in the steeplechase.

I asked him later about skipping that easy run and he said sometimes his body tells him it's not time to train. Kenyans understand their body better, I think. Whereas a Western athlete, if they are tired, would try to jam their way through it. I learned that from them and was a better athlete as a result.

The most dangerous part of a run is the start. The problems begin when we're feeling good. "Ah," we think, "I must be fully recovered."

We set off at a "reasonable" pace that's actually 5 or 10 percent faster than what's truly "easy." And the story always ends the same way. Those "not-quite-recovery" days start to add up to a big wall between the body and its complete recovery. Thus we find ourselves feeling blah and half-recovered on the runs that count—the planned longer and

---

26 "Olympian Then and Now: Bob Kennedy," *Runner's World,* June 4, 2012.

faster runs.

How can we know when we should take it easy, even if it means that we have to suppress our emotions and force ourselves to slow down?

We runners have two organs that can tell us, with great precision, when we aren't yet fully recovered. The first is our legs. The second is our heart.

Have you ever felt, after a hard run, that your physical heart was sore, tired, and bruised?

I have, many times. I take it as my body's clear signal that any further abuse will be dangerous. The heart isn't an organ to be toyed with. Former 10,000-meter world record holder Ron Clarke has an artificial heart. He blames the high-altitude 1968 Mexico City Olympics for the damage that made a transplant necessary.

A tired heart is invariably accompanied by tired emotions. A sure sign that we aren't fully recovered is a lack of enthusiasm. Until we're truly recovered, our legs, heart, and mind don't want to run. Our legs feel like slugs and our hearts are heavy and flat of feeling.

The tired-heart theory is supported by research reported in an article in *Scientific American*, "Ultra Marathons Might Be Ultra Bad for Your Heart." Researchers at the Mayo Clinic concluded that "excessive endurance exercise" may increase the risk of permanent heart damage and deadly cardiovascular events.

> "The researchers found that many of these athletes had temporarily elevated levels of substances that promote inflammation and cardiac damage. . . . And over time and with repeated exposure, these compounds can lead to scarring of the heart and its main arteries as well as to enlarged ventricles—all of which can in turn lead to

dangerous irregular heart beats (arrhythmia) and possibly sudden cardiac death."[27]

No wonder our hearts warn us with tired, depleted feelings that overdoing it is a mistake.

For many people, running a marathon or an ultra can be an expansive experience. It can help us develop will power, mental strength, and positive attitudes, and it builds a confidence that we can achieve our challenging goals.

But I've seen runners who'd long since stopped reaping the rewards and were plodding along regardless. It was clear that the sport had turned against them. It was eroding their health, happiness, and relationships. It was no longer expansive but contractive.

In my long-ago career as a sports photographer, I met a runner in his early 40s during the Double Dipsea race. He paused at the creek near Muir Woods where I was taking photos and wearily dowsed his head with water from the stream. He told me that on the two days before the race he'd completed hard 15-mile runs.

Later, *Runner's World* editor Joe Henderson told me that the runner's wife had left him, taking their children, because he'd chosen running over romance. Like most obsessed runners, he didn't look healthy or happy, just smugly worn-out.

When I entered the Western States 100, I reached the midpoint feeling unwell, uncertain if I should continue. I had repeated a short prayer all day, and as I approached the aid station at Michigan Bluff, I turned inward and told my

---

27. Katherine Harmon Courage, "Ultra Marathons Might Be Ultra Bad for Your Heart," *Scientific American* blog entry, June 4, 2012; http://blogs. scientificamerican.com/observations/2012/06/04/ultra-marathons-might-be-ultra-bad-for-your-heart/

spiritual teacher, "I'm not feeling good. I'm willing to go on, but please tell me what to do."

I heard his voice clearly. It said, "This is not healthy for your body."

I dropped out, not happily, but knowing I'd done the right thing.

When running reaches a point where it's no longer expansive, why bother? It's a simple question of weighing the costs and rewards. When the price of running is too high and the rewards are shrinking, maybe it's time to take stock and change direction.

17. FUN RUNNER:
A SANER WAY TO TRAIN

Abdi Abdirahman is a fun-loving guy. The four-time Olympian doesn't feel that running should be a drag.

Abdi was the subject of a *Wall Street Journal* profile that focused on his upbeat, relaxed disposition.

Abdirahman's coach, Dave Murray, believes it's this easy-going approach that has allowed him to avoid injuries, preserve his passion for running, and have a long career.[28]

I wonder if we couldn't benefit if we changed our focus, and avoided always living in some far-off paradise, always working for some future result, and instead tried to be more centered in the moment.

The Kenyan runners believe it's a defining difference between their approach and ours. Mike Kosgei, a former coach of Kenyan elites, uttered words for the ages:

When Europeans or Americans are running together, using stop watches and heart monitors, you can see for them it is a very serious matter, almost like work. Africans start running, mostly slow, and then they accelerate. For them, it is a kind of a game. You try to challenge the other. If you want to be successful, you have to enjoy your

---

28. Scott Cacciola, "Going for Gold—or Whatever," *Wall Street Journal*, May 15, 2012.

training. When you take it too seriously, it damages your thinking and puts you down. But if you go and say, okay, it is a game, man, let's do it, it's fun—then you will not use a lot of mental strength.[29]

As part of my self-therapy for chronic bronchitis, I do occasional juice fasts. In the second day of a fast, I decided to walk for an hour at a beautiful nature preserve by the San Francisco Bay.

It was a lovely spring morning. I felt like running, but didn't want to risk overdoing it during the fast. I reckoned I would just stroll and do whatever felt right.

I remembered something that Peter Snell said. In an interview with Rich Englehart, the three-time Olympic gold medalist recalled how he organized his speedwork while preparing for the 1964 Games where he won the 800m and 1500m. Rich lent me the recording of the interview, which I quote with his permission:

> Snell: That's how I sort of handled those sorts of long intervals, and making the transition between distance running and track running. I'd do something like 20 quarters in 65, and I had a full quarter jog in between. So actually that was like a 10-mile run.
>
> Q: Did you take a quarter jog between quarters?
>
> Snell: Mm-hm. Yup. And if I was doing work for the 800 meters, I would actually lie down and take a rest until I felt like doing another one.

I find that hilarious—"I would actually lie down and take a rest until I felt like doing another one."

It's so natural, human and real. It's the opposite of American Grim. As I ambled at the Baylands, I wondered if

---

29. Juerg Wirz, *Run to Win: Training Secrets of the Kenyan Runners* (Meyer & Meyer Verlag, 2006).

Snell's body had told him the best way to train.

In the midst of pursuits like running, which our culture tells us we should take terribly seriously, I believe there's room for a light heart. Ralph Waldo Emerson, as stern a cultural father figure as ever starched our national shirts, famously said, "Nothing great was ever accomplished without enthusiasm."

Must will power always be a grim affair?

The yoga sage, Paramhansa Yogananda, defined will power as "an increasingly smooth flow of energy and attention, directed toward a desired end."

What a mouthful! But it's packed with meaning. And it makes will power seem a lot more pleasant and achievable than the standard, frowning definitions.

Consider how it encompasses the five "tools of a runner":

Body = a "flow of energy"

Feeling = "desire"

Will = the "desired end" (a strong volition)

Mind = "attention"

Soul = the wisely chosen "desired end"

Of these tools, the heart is key. Nothing happens without "desire"—that is, enthusiasm. If we don't desire something badly enough, we simply won't bother. Desire, the longing of the heart, is the motor behind all of our worthwhile actions.

I enjoyed my walk at the Baylands. I ran when I felt my enthusiasm return, and stopped when it was no longer fun. Which, come to think of it, might be a reasonable way to train—for an Olympian like Abdi Abdirahaman, or a washed-up old crock like me.

18. WHAT RUNNERS WANT

In the movie *What Women Want*, Mel Gibson plays an advertising executive who uses women cynically.

As his boss remarks, he knows how to get what he wants from women, but he doesn't know how women think.

Gibson's character can't write ads for women, so his boss hires a woman, played by Helen Hunt, to create ads that will appeal to manufacturers of women's products.

Meanwhile, Gibson falls in a bathtub with a hair dryer and is shocked into unconsciousness. When he wakes up, he can hear what women are thinking.

It's a funny film, and surprisingly moving—I think because it shares an element with other stories that have the power to engage and inspire us: a protagonist who learns difficult lessons and becomes better than he was. As Gibson's character learns to see the world through women's eyes, his heart begins to open, and he feels moved to offer his female co-workers his friendship and support.

Thinking about the film, I recalled my run last weekend, and I reflected on how much more satisfying the experience of expanding awareness is, than its mirror-image in the movies.

I began the run feeling depressed and lethargic. I resolved that if inspiration and positive attitudes wouldn't come, I would do my best to create them.

I thought of Gary Fanelli. Gary is in his fifties and still

runs 10 miles under 55 minutes. Gary is famous for his positive attitude and off-beat sense of humor. As I mentioned earlier, when sports psychologists tested Gary, his scores on positive attitude were the highest they'd ever seen.

Ambling along, feeling depressed and directionless, I wondered how Gary manages to bring so much positive energy to his running. I decided that it's a question of perspective. Any experience can be positive, if we can understand it from the right angle. I resolved to fight free of my somber mood and pour my best energy into enjoying the day.

I was running on Mt. Tamalpais. After stopping at the Pantoll ranger station to fill my water bottles, I took a wrong turn and faced a decision: I could go overland, straight up a long, incredibly steep, grassy hill, or turn around and take a much longer route back to the trail.

Inching painfully up the slope, knees to nose, I panted with silent laughter. But the energy I generated was the cure for my blues. Emerging onto the trail, I felt renewed, my spirits restored.

The ridge above Pantoll is one of the loveliest places on earth. Green meadows flow over rolling hillsides punctuated by groves of evergreen and oak, down to the blue Pacific 2000 feet below.

The ridgetop trails were wonderfully harmonious and serene. Couples were seated on rocky outcrops under windblown cypresses, absorbing the amazing views. On a grassy knoll, a native Australian played a didgeridoo for friends sprawled in a circle on the grass.

I paused to take pictures with my little camera, then started the long descent. I wore my heart monitor, and for the umpteenth time I was able to confirm that science, spirit, and the runner's art are completely in accord. I kept my heart rate in the "harmony zone," while I practiced inward chanting and let my heart open to nature's welcoming embrace. It was a lovely afternoon.

The four-mile descent was jarring. But with an easy pace and a joyous mental attitude, I managed to stay in the harmony zone. I'm learning the joy of finding the place inside where body and mind, feeling, will, and soul coalesce.

Back to the movies. In the arts, it's almost a sure thing, given adequate craft, that if the artist's vision is expansive, human hearts will respond. We're attracted to movies and books that show us paths to more awareness and joy, just as we're attracted to sports heroes who point the direction toward our own higher potential.

The way to get more happiness is by loving more, serving more, living with greater energy, growing in wisdom, letting go of petty self-importance, and embracing a greater Self. That's the formula. How well it succeeds in the arts depends, in part, on the skill of the actors and director, but much more on the wisdom of the artist.

Shakespeare must have expanded his heart greatly, to be able to write about life's grand themes. Lesser authors may be unable to hold the same broad vision, but they can be expansive at their level. An advertising executive learns to think like a woman, and by expanding his heart, he becomes a better man.

19. RUNNERS AND DEMONS

P. G. Wodehouse, the English humorist, observed that there are two kinds of American businessman. One is the hale and hearty fellow who'll slap you on the back, shove a drink in your hand, and tell you two off-color jokes before you can sit down.

The other is the kind who worships at the shrine of the dollar and sits grimly at the head of the table, his glowering eyes radiating disapproval of everything and everyone.

I've known runners who seemed constitutionally incapable of taking the sport lightly. They were serious about it all the time. For them, it was hideously important to wear the right clothing, create the right schedules, and track the behavior of their hearts on a computer.

Every moment of each workout had to be serious. When they weren't grimly doing quarter-mile repeats, they were grimly talking about their stock options. They were runners who wanted desperately to *get ahead*, and for whom morality and sport were thickly intertwined.

Joseph Epstein, a former editor of *The American Scholar*, wrote an amusing essay on "virtuecracy." The virtuecrat is the type of person, he explained, often found in newspaper editorial offices, who compulsively rates people on his private scale of virtue.

The virtuecrat runner is prepared to judge your shoes,

your race PRs, the length of your hair, the age of your car, your girlfriend's looks, and your income, all at a glance. You'll never be able to run *with* a virtuecrat, because he'll always be compelled to stay one step ahead.

It's an approach to running that, on the brief occasions I've tried it, tripped me badly. Just yesterday, I ran 20 minutes and found myself, in that short time, falling into the trap of virtuecracy, measuring my virtue as a runner and feeling that I was sadly deficient.

I had taken several days off and felt that I should be rested and able to run fast. But I felt crappy, and I judged myself for it. There drifted into my mind the dark thought: "This is inadequate. You've done something wrong. You've made some mistake. You are a *Bad Runner.*"

The quality of the run was destroyed. If I had accepted reality and slowed to a jog, falling in with the crappy spirit of the run and drawing maximum amusement and enjoyment from it, I believe I'd have gone home with a smile.

In fact, that's what's wrong with mixing virtuecracy and running—it kills the fun.

I remember a dried-up Grim American runner who, catching sight of my battered '82 Honda Civic before the start of a 30K race, curled his lip in supercilious scorn. Get it together, his sere and wrinkled mug said—you shouldn't bring such a crappy car to a race. We are yuppies. You don't belong.

The Civic was a wonderful car. *Pepito* got great gas mileage and had no extra doo-dads that ever needed fixing. It was beneath the contempt of car thieves, parked like a SmartCar, and expressed my monkish view of life, based on simplicity and detachment from worldly things.

Yesterday I watched a wonderful documentary, filmed by

an Irish TV network, about Brother Colm O'Connell, the Catholic monk who started the Kenyan running revolution, and who still coaches dozens of elites.

A notable feature of the Kenyans' training is that it is *relaxed*. If a day goes badly, and the energy isn't there for a long, hard session, they accept it as the natural ebb and flow of life and run accordingly.

Mike Kosgei, the Kenyan national coach for 15 years (1985–95, 2001–04), says:

After having a bad workout, a European might think about it for many days. It can really affect him, And he might lose days of good training. A Kenyan will forget about it immediately. If I was not strong today, I will be next time. (From *Run to Win: The Training Secrets of the Kenyan Runners*, by Juerg Wirz.)

From the American Grim perspective, these words are unacceptable—they're irresponsible. Yet I wonder if they don't express the spirit of running as nature intended.

After all, the ultimate reason we run isn't for the product or the process, but to find happiness and avoid suffering. At any rate, I enjoy my running most when I can free myself from the grim virtue-judging demons that try to whip me from inside.

20. EXPANSIVE SPORTS

It's been a wonderful year for sports books.

The last 12 months have seen the publication of three classics: Bill Rodgers's *Marathon Man*, Alberto Salazar's *14 Minutes*, and Phil Jackson's *Eleven Rings: The Soul of Success*.

A strong theme running throughout these books is that they're about expansive sports—the notion that positive energy, positive attitudes, and a focus on individual improvement lead to success.

Jackson's account of his remarkable NBA career as a coach and player takes us inside his relationships with superstars Michael Jordan, Scottie Pippen, Kobe Bryant, Dennis Rodman, Shaquille O'Neal, and many others. His memoir doesn't have a boring page. It's wonderful.

How did Jackson persuade so many sports stars to cooperate—to become warrior-brothers instead of prima donnas? More on Jackson in a moment.

In an earlier chapter, I proposed that sports championships are won by those who embrace expansive attitudes. Examples from today's sports pages include the Seattle Seahawks, the Nike Oregon Project, and the African elites.

Soon after reading *Eleven Rings*, I chanced upon a wonderful article by Alyssa Roenigk in *ESPN The Magazine*. In "Lotus Pose on Two," Roenigk describes how coach Pete Carroll transformed the Seattle Seahawks into the best team in the NFL.

His [Carroll's] dream was to fundamentally change the way players are coached. The timeworn strategy is, of course, to be a hard-ass—think Bear Bryant banning water breaks, Vince Lombardi screaming and yelling, Mike Rice throwing basketballs at players' heads, Nick Saban berating his team on the sideline. Carroll craved a chance to reimagine the coaching role in the NFL. "I wanted to find out if we went to the NFL and really took care of guys, really cared about each and every individual, what would happen?"

What happened is that on December 13, 2012, the Seahawks demolished the San Francisco Forty-Niners, their most dangerous rivals, by a score of 40-13.

The lopsided victory doesn't begin to tell the story. "Demolished" is too weak a word. *Crushed, annihilated, obliterated, shamed, humiliated, destroyed, waxed, astonished, devastated.*

The Seahawks looked like tigers playing with mice. And the Forty-Niners were a very good team—at the end of the season they came within four yards of winning the Super Bowl.

Great coaches realize that a key to success is caring for the individual athlete. If the players are unhappy, feel disrespected, or are divided, the team will have greatly reduced chances of succeeding. Contractive attitudes divert energy or kill it.

Of course, the energy of the team begins with the energy of the individual player. Good coaches know that every player is unique and needs individual mentoring. Phil Jackson, in *Eleven Rings*:

My approach was always to relate to each player as a whole person, not just as a cog in the basketball machine. That meant pushing him to discover what distinct qualities he could bring to the game beyond taking shots and making passes. How much courage did he have? Or resilience? What about character under fire? Many players I've coached didn't look special on paper, but in the process of creating a role for themselves they grew into formidable champions. Derek Fisher is a prime example. He began as a backup point guard for the Lakers with average foot speed and shooting skills. But he worked tirelessly and transformed himself into an invaluable clutch performer and one of the best leaders I've ever coached.

Pete Carroll found success by the same principles. The ESPN article relates how he banned yelling and swearing at players, and insisted that players end media interviews with a polite thank-you.

The Seahawks coaches closely monitor their players' lives—from their sleep patterns, to their personal goals, and how they're able to deal with stress. "Depressed? Worried about a loved one? Sick pet? The staff wants to hear about it." The coaches are expected to adapt to the system, too. Former Raiders coach Tom Cable, known as a hothead while in Oakland, describes how working with Carroll transformed the way he relates with players. Instead of screaming, he's now focused on helping them fix their weaknesses.

Another lesson shared by these three excellent books is the value of being centered in the moment. Phil Jackson:

> At the start of every season I always encouraged players to focus on the journey rather than the goal. What matters most is playing the game the right way and having the courage to grow, as human beings as well as basketball players. When you do that, the ring takes care of itself.

A final lesson is that external rewards don't last. The satisfactions of a sub-3-hour marathon, or even an NBA championship, will fade over time. But the joys of the moment are always available. Phil Jackson says he's no longer moved much by winning trophies; that what counts now is helping young players "tap into the magic" that comes by focusing, heart and soul, on shared goals.

During the Niners game, Seahawk quarterback Russell Wilson's poise was ethereal. He seemed to smile with an inner peace. Wilson is a fan of the team's obligatory meditation practices. Pete Carroll believes that meditation helps the players stay calm and efficient under pressure, and able to ground themselves during the chaos of a game. Offensive tackle Russell Okung is a fan: "Meditation is as important as lifting weights and being out here on the field for practice"

Throughout Jackson's career, especially his first years with the Chicago Bulls, he was teased for his new-age methods, including his attempts to get his players to meditate. Jackson felt that his Zen practice had helped him be a better coach. Michael Jordan wasn't much interested, but Steve Kerr and others felt that meditation helped them.

Bill Rodgers' autobiography, *Marathon Man: My 26.2-Mile Journey from Unknown Grad Student to the Top of the Running World,* may be the best elite runner's bio since Ron Clarke's *The Unforgiving Minute* (1966).

Rodgers won Boston and New York four times each. He was a natural, a guy the other stars were in awe of, for his beautiful running form, his tremendous talent, and his boundless energy.

Marathon Man is rich with insider stories from the glory years of US running, told in "Boston Billy's" genial style. Rodgers doesn't try to impress us with his distant successes.

But he's an unabashed flag-bearer for his approach to training and racing. A lesson he hopes we'll take from his book and his life is that training is most successful when it's fun. Rodgers believes enjoyment comes by running hard and cultivating mental relaxation.

I think we run best when we are calm and relaxed; at least, that's what I've found.... I have a better idea of what strategy to employ; I can hear what my body is telling me.

Rodgers didn't hammer himself daily in training—most miles were run at a moderate (for him) 7:00 to 6:30 pace. He trained almost exclusively on a 1.5-mile loop around a small lake. Not being able to enjoy nature while he ran was unthinkable. He felt that natural surroundings contributed to his success, by helping him keep a positive attitude.

Rodgers doesn't gloss over his years as a penniless grad student who lost his way and sought refuge in cigarettes and booze. The down time provides a dark backdrop for the ascending light of his return to running. Plodding through life with heavy feelings of depression and meaninglessness, Rodgers ultimately found redemption in his work with the mentally ill, and in his relationship with his wife, Ellen.

Rodgers had ADHD (attention deficit hyperactivity disorder). It manifested as a spaciness that was part of what made him loveable. Another upside is that it helped his running, paradoxically enabling him to become utterly focused while running.

The atmosphere among the top American runners during Rodgers's prime years, in the early 1970s, was informal and collegial. He believes it's a mistake to dismiss the value of that closeness.

If you want to see the tight club mentality of the seventies running boom, you need to travel to Kenya and

Ethiopia. It's no surprise they now dominate the distance events.

Alberto Salazar's *14 Minutes: A Running Legend's Life and Death and Life* is a bit of an odd duck, viewed against the books by Rodgers and Jackson. The title refers to the day Salazar collapsed and his heart stopped beating for fourteen minutes.

Salazar's Catholic faith provides a framework for his life story. While some readers may prefer their sports heroes to be agnostic, or tight-lipped about their beliefs, Salazar's faith helped transform him from a maniacally driven marathoner to a coach whose concern is what's best for his runners.

Salazar is emerging as one of history's great running coaches. Today, it seems that being accepted by the Nike Oregon Project is a near-guarantor of success. Mo Farah and Galen Rupp, coached by Salazar, won two golds (Farah) and a silver (Rupp)—at the London Olympics in 2012.

Salazar's faith helped him recognize that life is larger than running. It's a lesson that Jackson, Rodgers, and Carroll learned in their own ways. Expanding our awareness to include the welfare of others gives our lives meaning. It lays an optimal foundation for success. Salazar:

Compared to the contributions of others, running around a track faster than a rival, or running from point A to point B ahead of another man, doesn't amount to much. To the degree that those races pointed me toward a deeper faith, however, or inspired others to evaluate their lives in a more meaningful light, they have value. I had been gradually building toward that insight for years, but my near-death experience in 2007 drove it home indelibly.

21. FATIGUE AND INTUITION

I don't know how runners survive without using their intuition.

At the start of our careers, we're counseled to "listen to the body." I doubt many beginners take the advice seriously. I certainly didn't. Yet it's one of life's most insistent lessons: *learn to listen! Pay attention!* Mostly, I reckon we learn it the hard way.

In time, experience tells us that each moment of a run can be meaningful, rich with information. To tap that inner wisdom, all we have to do is hear what the run is trying to tell us.

On a recent long run, I experienced the value of intuition for the umpteenth time.

I felt strangely tired—it wasn't the fatigue of overtraining, but an elderly, frail feeling. (I'm 73.) My legs lacked pep, and my heart and lungs felt weak, unable to work hard.

When I tried to parse the problem with logic, I came up with a big, fat zero.

I had done all the right things. I'd taken carbs, water, and electrolytes. After the run, I drank Recoverite. Yet I continued to feel blah, although overtraining seemed unlikely.

I decided to turn off logic and consult my intuition. I asked for guidance, and the answer came. I felt intuitively, with the heart's sure knowing, that what my body needed was *grease*.

When I got home, I made another Recoverite drink with goat's milk, frozen strawberries, and rice syrup. Then I ate goat cheese with crackers. An hour later, I still felt cored-out and ravenous. When I consulted my intuition again, the answer was: *more grease!*

I fried two veggie burgers in four tablespoons of coconut oil. It was perfect, profoundly satisfying. Within minutes I knew that it was what my body needed. An hour later, my energy had returned and my mood was upbeat. I felt whole again. The next day, I was more recovered than after any long run in months.

Later, I remembered something I'd read in tennis great Pete Sampras's autobiography, *A Champion's Mind: Lessons from a Life in Tennis*.

Sampras was very disciplined about his diet. He wouldn't let junk food enter the temple of his body. At one point, he began feeling a mysterious fatigue that caused him to lose an important match. When he consulted his intuition, it gave him the same message I received: *Grease!* Sampras ate some appropriately greasy food, and his energy quickly returned.

Lesson learned: don't be spellbound by the "rules" of training, but be ready to adjust them in response to your body's actual needs.

22. MINIMALISM: EXTERNAL AND INTERNAL

One kind of minimalism is easy and costs a bundle.

The other kind is cheap, but more difficult.

There's external minimalism—stripping down our gear in search of a simpler, more primitive kind of enjoyment. It involves buying expensive "minimalist" shoes, mini-packs, and trendy trips to run with the Tarahumara in northern Mexico.

Then there's inner minimalism—calming restless thoughts and feelings in search of a simple heart.

Which minimalism delivers the best rewards?

A problem with outward minimalism is that stripped-down gear doesn't change *us*.

To experience minimalism at its core, a runner needs to move the focus inside, away from funny-looking shoes and other externals.

My first brush with minimalism came in 1968, the year I started running. I ran on the beach, barefoot and shirtless, feeling connected in spirit with people who lived a thousand years before and ran in primal simplicity, for the sheer joy.

As my endurance grew, I did longer runs, keeping them as simple as possible. In the early 1970s, I lived in Mill Valley, across the Golden Gate from San Francisco. On weekends I would drive my '72 VW Bug to the City for long runs in

Golden Gate Park.

I was fanatically simple. I hid the car keys under a tire, not wanting to carry even those tiny reminders of civilization. I lugged no food or water and didn't wear a watch—I ran in shorts and shoes, that was all. I loved those nature-boy runs of 14 to 18 miles.

In time, I graduated to ultramarathons. I loved the feeling, late in a 50-miler, of being reduced to a very simple, frail old person, tottering along in a temple of silence—my mind no longer capable of chattering, my emotional reactions muted, my spirit humbled to a childlike serenity.

At one point, I ran five 50Ks in six weeks, yet none of those shorter runs could equal the simplifying power of 50 miles.

My last ultra was a solo 50-miler, done as a school fundraiser. At 5 a.m. on a spring morning in 2003, I dipped a finger in San Francisco Bay, and 12½ hours later I stretched my tired legs in the ocean at Pescadero Beach and let the waves wash over them.

By then, minimalism had become a comfortable habit. Aside from fuel and water in a small backpack, my only aid was a gallon of water stashed in the bushes up on the ridge, and a bottle of juice purchased from a roadside stand.

I've always loved simplicity. I find that stripped-down gear helps me achieve that wonderful primal feeling, but stripping away restless thoughts takes me deeper.

Becoming simple inside is seldom easy. I spent 20 years testing ways to still my restless mind, with little success. It became much easier when I realized that the key lies in stilling the heart.

My spiritual teacher knew that I had serious issues with mental restlessness. Yet he never urged me to meditate more.

Soon after I came to him, I was meditating as much as 5½ hours a day, and not getting anywhere. I was grinding it out. I asked him how I could develop more heart quality.

He said, "That is your single greatest need." He said, "You should chant."

Wanting to be honest, I said, "But, Sir, I don't think I'm a chanter by nature." He said matter-of-factly, "Well, you should." It was the closest he ever came to giving me a direct order, and it was merely a suggestion that I was free to accept or ignore.

He said, "It's dry when you slog along with techniques."

In time, I discovered that opening my heart helped my meditations tremendously, and it helped my running, too.

I relish the experience of running in a "zone" state, where my mind becomes still and running is an effortless flow. As I found ways to harmonize my heart, I discovered that the inner silence came more easily.

I was most successful when I filled my heart with feelings of love, kindness, and compassion. Enjoyment was the key. When my heart was happy, my mind gladly rested in those feelings.

The more I practiced, the more I realized that getting into the zone isn't a question of reaching outward, but of falling into a timeless place in the heart.

23. THE KEY TO RUNNING SUCCESS

I live in Silicon Valley, cradle of exciting technologies.

Years ago, I discovered a way to predict, with a high degree of accuracy, if a tech company would succeed or fail. This simple principle works equally well for predicting success in running.

Consider a company that I worked for in the late 1990s and early 2000s.

The moment I walked in the door, I was inspired by the company's technology. They made software that helped software developers do their jobs.

Helping others expands our hearts. It's an enjoyable experience. The company's products felt good.

Yet, despite its expansive technology, the company was riddled with contractive attitudes.

Honest people didn't stay there long. They were fired or they quit. I was never so grateful as when a particularly arrogant manager stopped giving me consulting work.

It was a paradox. The product was expansive, but the management was bafflingly contractive.

After he left, a friend who'd been an executive at the company told me how the employees would routinely lie to each other. I witnessed how the managers bullied and micromanaged their subordinates.

My friend was a principled man. When he left to start

his own consultancy, we met for lunch. He told me how the company had imploded during the dot-com bust. The once-mighty enterprise, which had lavished money on ego-gratifying projects like sponsoring a sports team, was now an empty shell.

Interestingly, the company's wonderful technology survived, finding a more expansive home at Hewlett-Packard.

Long ago in India, wise men asked a simple question: "What do people want?" The answer they arrived at was both simple and profound. Observing the human scene with calm objectivity, they realized that what everyone in the world is seeking, behind the multiplicity of their stated motives, is to experience greater happiness, and avoid suffering.

The sages realized that the way to accomplish these two ends is by expanding our awareness.

"Expansion equals happiness." I find this simple principle is the only guidance I need for my training. No matter if I'm doing long runs, speedwork, tempo runs, or strength training, if I do it in a way that generates expansive feelings, I thrive. But if my training feels disharmonious, contractive, or subtly "wrong," I get poor results and suffer. As we saw in chapters 5 and 6, positive, expansive feelings make our hearts beat in a smooth, harmonious rhythm that enables it to work more efficiently at any pace.

As an old guy, I can no longer train hard as often as when I was young. Because I enjoy those infrequent hard days, I take care to protect them, by trying to run expansively on the easy days.

This has two happy benefits. Running the right way on the light days makes those easy runs very enjoyable, and it lets me run faster on my rare hard days.

"Happiness." "Joy." These are my training partners.

24. A RUNNER'S PATH

Gerry Lindgren still holds the high school indoor records for 3000m and 2 miles (8:06.3 and 8:40.0), more than 50 years after he ran those amazing times in 1964.

Gerry's training in high school was jaw-dropping. Few teens consistently run 150 to 250 miles per week, as he did.

Lindgren still loves to run. His memories are laced with high spirits:

We didn't keep track of how many miles we ran back then. We just ran. If you LOVE to run with the kind of passion I have for running, you will understand this. Running was my mode of transportation.

The interview where these comments appeared, in *Youth Runner* magazine[30], was an enjoyable read. That is, until the end, where Gerry uttered words that should never have been published in a magazine for aspiring young runners.

Everyone dies whether one is good in their lifetime or evil in their lifetime. So virtue has no payback. Life is meaningless. When you die, you die! . . . We are here for the benefit, happiness, and welfare of a new reality; a new direction.

Gerry's words are positive in their overall effect. He believes we should radiate goodness every moment of our lives. That's the kind of guy Gerry is. In its entry on him,

---

30. "Gerry Lindgren Interview," *Youth Runner Magazine*, January 12, 2011.

Wikipedia says:

Lindgren has reiterated his belief in "Karma" as a large factor in his running success. He claims, "Karma comes from serving other people instead of serving yourself. I found that if I could serve other people without them knowing about it I could grow Karma faster," and that this would lead to success on the track.

But—"Virtue has no payback?" And "Life is meaningless?"

Gerry was speaking off the cuff. Perhaps his thoughts reflected a passing mood. Regardless, the editors of *Youth Runner* should be pelted with lavender buds and dipped up to their necks in lilac water for allowing those nihilistic words in print.

It's the only way I can think of to rid them of the stench from the rotting corpses of Jean-Paul Sartre and his fellow nihilists, which continues to stink-up the brains of students in our colleges and universities.

Alternatively, they should be sentenced to read J. Donald Walters's outstanding book, *Out of the Labyrinth—For Those Who Want to Believe, But Can't*. It's the most powerful antidote to Jean-Paul's putrid *pensées* I've found.

Life isn't meaningless. Neither is running—sourpuss French *philosophes* notwithstanding. I trot forth as evidence a simple notion from *Out of the Labyrinth* that has immediate practical applications for runners. It's called "directional relativity."

Consider the training of the African elites. It's beyond my comprehension. Yet I find that I can practice the same *principles* by which they train, scaled to the talents of a 73-year-old bog-snorkeler like me.

Haile Gebrselassie and I will never train together. What's healthy for the great Ethiopian would murder me. Yet we're training in the same general direction, toward increasing fitness, health, and joy. That's directional relativity.

Directional relativity is how life works. And it drives a stake in the heart of the fashionable Sartrean notion that life is meaningless.

It also dispels any number of false notions about running—for example, the idea that runners who share the same goal—say, a 3:30 marathon—should train the same.

The worst books on running say: "If you want to run 3:30, here are six months of daily training schedules that will get you there."

Most runners today would recognize that kind of advice as drivel. Training isn't about following a rigid system. It's about choosing proven *principles* and juggling the million varied details with skill.

The "best" training changes daily—nay, every hour and minute. When your body is tired, or your Achilles hurts, or you've eaten something that disagreed with you, or you've slept poorly, or the weather is horrible—the best training is what moves you in the right *direction*, without breaking your body or killing your joy.

In this realistic scheme of things, no training is ever wasted. Even our slowest runs have value, so long as they move us forward, toward more fitness and fulfillment.

Ultramarathoners have a wonderful acronym: "RFP." It means Relentless Forward Progress. When you're halfway through a 50- or 100-miler, and you're feeling awful, it means that you're a winner if you just keep moving forward, even if you have to crawl.

Gerry got it partly right. Life holds the promise of great joy—a joy that comes when we expand our awareness through our body, heart, will, mind, and soul.

25. ANSWERS

Where can runners turn when they have difficult questions?

Science? Science is notorious for revising or overturning its favorite theories every few years. In the introduction, I relate how exercise physiologists believed for 80 years that lactic acid caused the "burn" during hard running. Then lactic acid was revealed to be a fuel for the working muscles.

Another problem with exercise science is that it describes broad, average behaviors. But it offers little help for the individual runner.

Where can we go to find the answers we need?

Famous coaches? There are lots of them. They aren't all equally wise. And good luck hiring one.

For my money, Lydiard was the wisest, most trustworthy coach of all time, simply because he proved his ideas in the laboratory of his own training—and he proved them over and over with the world-class athletes who set records by following his methods.

I got blasted when I posted an unwelcome comment on the *Runner's World* forum. I said, approximately, "God help the beginning runner who comes here for answers. He'll get so many conflicting replies, he'll be thoroughly bewildered. And many of the answers will be little more than personal opinions tossed off without attention to the runner's unique needs."

Judging from the violence of the reaction, people hated to hear that. Yet I believe it's true. I wasn't trying to be provocative. I was describing my own experience, years before, when I posted my own beginner-type questions online. I got such a bewildering variety of answers that I didn't know which way to turn.

I had better luck when I began to consult my intuition. Specifically, when I asked my intuition what I should do, and listened carefully in my heart for the answer.

Occasionally, rarely, the answers came in spectacular fashion.

When I began training for marathons and ultras, I got seriously overtrained. I was running long every weekend, and I was running the long runs straight through without walking breaks. I was often sick with colds and diarrhea, and I was tired all the time.

Desperate for answers, I was driving on the freeway through Grass Valley, praying to know what to do, when I heard an intuitive voice—it was my spiritual teacher. It said, "Go see Jim Walker."

Jim was a well-known runner who worked at a local sporting goods store. Jim had run 112 marathons, the Western States 100 four times, the American River 50 eight times, and the notorious 135-mile Badwater race across Death Valley in midsummer.

In my prayer, I said, "But Jim's boss gives me the evil eye whenever I go in the store and start yakking with him."

Again the intuitive voice said: "Go see Jim Walker."

When I got to the store, Jim's boss was gone. I told Jim how I'd been training, and he draped an arm over a clothes rack and proceeded to lecture me on how to do my long runs, taking walking breaks and never running too fast or long.

Training is complex. Often we can't find the answers we need because we can't know all the factors involved. What's causing this heel pain? A "scientific" answer might include minute descriptions of bone, cartilage, cell metabolism, blood flow, pronation, shoe construction, running form—on and on. All with lots of "maybes" and "perhapses" thrown in. It might take days to ferret out all the factors and weigh them in the scale of logic and reason before we can identify a tentative cure.

I've had better luck consulting a power that knows my needs and has my best interests at heart.

26. BILL ARIS'S TRUTH: HOW HEARTFELT RUNNING MAKES CHAMPIONS

Nobody believes Bill Aris.

People ask Bill, over and over, how his Fayetteville-Manlius High School (NY) cross country girls' team has managed to win Nike Cross Nationals eight times. (NXN is the de facto high school national team championships.)

Bill graciously shares his methods. He patiently explains how he trains his runners. And other coaches suspect he's *signifyin'*.

Surely he's pulling their tails. At least, he's got to be holding something back.

Coaches fall off their chairs when Bill explains that he spends relatively little time designing workouts.

"I spend 80 percent of my time on psychological and emotional considerations of each kid," Aris said. "I put 20 percent of my time in designing the training," he said. "I spend most of my time thinking about and trying to get to the heart and soul of each kid, to both inspire them and to understand them. I'm always trying to figure out what keys unlock what doors to get them to maximize their potential."[31]

---

31. Tom Leo and Donnie Webb, "The Secret to F-M's Success: There Is No Secret," Syracuse.com, December 10, 2010. http://highschoolsports.syracuse.com/news/article/4542182549305228511/the-secret-to-f-m-cross-countrys-success-there-is-no-secret/

Other coaches believe there's no way Aris can produce national champions, year after year, without huge numbers of kids trying out for the team, and without recruiting.

In fact, Fayetteville-Manlius has 1500–2000 students, yet just 25 runners show up each fall for cross country. And Aris doesn't have to recruit, because his methods turn talented kids into champions.

The boys' teams won NXN in 2014, and they've placed second several times, plus a third and fourth.

To put that in perspective, it's an enormous honor to be invited to NXN. Scoring consistently in the top five puts the F-M boys in the stratosphere of the nation's high school teams.

At the library recently, I picked up an outstanding book. At first glance, former U.S. Navy Captain D. Michael Abrashoff's *It's Your Ship: Management Techniques from the Best Damn Ship in the Navy* would appear to have little to do with training high school girls and boys. But Bill Aris and Mike Abrashoff are a lot alike. They're renegade thinkers, in professions where the safe path to career advancement is doing things the way they've always been done.

Abrashoff describes what happened when the Navy assigned him command of a troubled ship with bottom-of-the-barrel efficiency ratings.

In the Navy, officers are expected to get ahead or get out. If they aren't being promoted on a regular basis, they risk being seen as damaged goods, and shunted into posts where they can't taint the careers of other officers.

It's a system that breeds a paranoid management style, where the highest priority is not looking bad. It encourages officers to micromanage their subordinates to get results that will look good on their resumes.

That approach has terrible consequences for morale. When Abrashoff took over *Benfold*, most of the crew members told him they couldn't wait to leave the ship and get out of the Navy.

What Captain Abrashoff did was amazing. I laughed, smiled, and occasionally wiped a tear as I read. Abrashoff decided to apply the lessons he'd learned during a two-year stint as aide to Secretary of Defense William J. Perry. He would put the crew's welfare first—as Bill Aris does with his runners.

Abrashoff interviewed each of *Benfold's* 310 crew members personally, asking them about their backgrounds, their life goals, what they hoped to get out of their time in the Navy, and what they felt was wrong with the Navy's way of doing things.

Above all, he invited their suggestions for improving procedures in their departments. And he implemented their ideas, even if it meant bending regulations.

Within six months, *Benfold* was winning at-sea exercises against ships with stronger reputations.

Abrashoff adopted a simple guiding principle:

"I decided that on just about everything I did, my standard should be simply whether or not it felt right. You can never go wrong if you do 'the right thing.' . . .

If it feels right, smells right, tastes right, it's almost surely the right thing—and you will be on the right track.

"If that doesn't sound very profound or sophisticated, in the Navy, in business, and in life, it really is as simple as that."

Let's add "in sports training." We *know* when we're doing the right training—it feels right. And we know when we're screwing up—it feels subtly wrong. It's simple. Do the right thing and your training goes well, and you enjoy it.

Few believed Abrashoff's expansive leadership style would work—until *Benfold* began to earn a reputation as "the best damn ship in the Navy."

Assigned to the Persian Gulf during the second Gulf War, *Benfold* became the go-to ship when commanders needed things done quickly and correctly. When other captains wanted to improve their ships' performance, they visited *Benfold* and talked with Abrashoff and his crew.

It's an incredibly inspiring story. And the principles behind USS *Benfold's* success are the same as those that led the teams of Fayetteville-Manlius to nine national championships.

In my working life, I occasionally help Donovan R. Greene, PhD, a successful industrial psychologist. Companies hire Don to identify executives who can help them improve their corporate culture. A habit that many of the best candidates share is "managing by walking around" (MBWA).

That's what Mike Abrashoff did. He spent hours in each of *Benfold's* departments, learning about its functions and where it fit within the ship's operations. He got to know the crew and invited their thoughts on how they could do their jobs better.

He empowered the crew members to make changes. He respected them and tapped their creativity, knowledge, and enthusiasm. Morale soared and success came quickly.

It was similar to how Bill Aris manages his cross country teams.

Coaches don't believe Bill Aris, because he doesn't tell them what they want to hear. They want to hear: "I get results by hard-nosed methods. I work my runners' tails off, and I'm not above recruiting if I don't get caught. We do huge mileage in summer, and I won't tell you about our speedwork, because that would be revealing too much. It's all in the numbers."

When sports scientists from America and Europe travel to Africa to study the Kenyan elite runners, they bring along their little measuring sticks. They measure the Kenyans' leg lengths, muscle elasticity, calf and thigh dimensions. And they weigh and analyze what they eat—how much carbohydrate, fat, and protein. They study how many miles they run, and how hard. And they write it all down in a little notebook full of numbers.

Few of them ask the Kenyans about their hopes and dreams. Yet if you ask the Kenyans to explain the difference between themselves and their American and European counterparts, they don't mention numbers. They talk about qualities of the heart—not heart volume and such-like science, but the *feelings* of the heart.

They explain that they run based on inner feeling—that they take joy in running together, and that if their bodies don't feel ready to run they'll pack it in and go home, whereas an American runner might force himself through the workout, haunted by a need to "make the numbers." The Kenyans know that their bodies will tell them when it's okay to run hard.

They talk about how the U.S. runners are so *serious* about their training, how obsessed they are with numbers and technology, and how it's all geared toward some feverishly imagined tomorrow. Meanwhile, the Kenyans are intent on maximizing the joys of *today*.

Captain Abrashoff did a simple thing on *Benfold*—he created a happy ship. Other ships' officers and crew members were soon looking for excuses to visit *Benfold*, to be uplifted and infected by its upbeat mood.

That's the secret of Bill Aris's success, and it isn't complicated. Aris creates happy teams. How? By getting to know his runners and helping them realize their dreams. That kind of caring creates loyalty, enthusiasm, and success, whether on a missile destroyer or a cross country course.

When Abrashoff left *Benfold*, he studied surveys conducted by the Navy to discover why people weren't re-enlisting. Surprisingly, low pay was the fifth reason. "The top reason was not being treated with respect or dignity; second was being prevented from making an impact on the organization; third, not being listened to; and fourth, not being rewarded with more responsibility."

Abrashoff worked tirelessly to reverse these trends aboard *Benfold*. He wouldn't tolerate attitudes that would risk creating a bossy, feudal culture rampant with resentful feelings. Every crew member's contribution was to be considered important, and they were to be made aware of their value to the ship. By treating his crew as if they mattered, and giving them freedom to shine, Abrashoff built the best damn ship in the Navy—just as Aris built the nation's best cross country teams.

Six months after his departure, *Benfold* earned *the highest grade in the history of the Pacific Fleet* on the Navy's Combat Systems Readiness Review.

Abrashoff tells story after story of how he transformed the culture of his ship, one detail at a time. It's very moving. Ultimately the "method" can be boiled down to a simple principle: the best approach to organizational change is the one that creates the greatest fulfillment for each individual.

"Every year, I look at every kid in our group," Aris said. "Number one, I try to find out what's in their mind and in their hearts. How high is up, in other words. From there I build a training program around that."

By building up the individual runner, says high school running journalist Marc Bloom, Bill Aris has created a unique culture.

"In all my 40-plus years (being involved with cross country) I don't think I've seen anything this extraordinary, at least on the high school level. . . . If you look at professionals it's like looking at the Kenyans and the Ethiopians. On the high school level, F-M is so far better than anyone else.

"You say how do they do it?" Bloom added. "You can look at the physiological aspect and the running, but there is also a cultural foundation to it. It's a different society. It's a different attitude."[32]

It's a culture that engenders good feelings in each runner and within the team. Aris persuades his runners to tap the joys of training for something larger than themselves.

"When our kids train and or race, they do so for each other rather than competing against each other. When one releases themselves from the limiting constraints of individual achievement alone, new worlds open up in terms of group AND individual potential and its fulfillment. . . . Each is capable of standing on their own, but when working together so much more is accomplished both for the group and individual. The whole is greater than the sum of its parts basically, nothing new here.

"Next, I would suggest the notion of contribution rather than participation. By this I mean that each kid on our team has an opportunity to contribute to the overall good rather than to merely participate in the process. In this way, regardless of whatever level on the team a kid may be in terms of ability or competitive success, each

32. *Ibid.*

strives to see themselves as giving something worthwhile of themselves to improve our process, rather than to merely participate or take from the program. Simply put, giving versus taking. All of this is program-wide, inclusive of both the boys and girls I coach."[33]

Why aren't people more receptive to these radical but thoroughly tested ideas? Why are so few listening?

Perhaps Mark Allen, six-time winner of the Hawaii Ironman Triathlon, has the answer.

Allen was a hard-charging trainer, a former All-American swimmer at UC San Diego. Swimmers do intense interval workouts, and when Allen became a triathlete he trained full-out, all the time, whether he was running, riding, or swimming. Yet, year after year, he fell just short of winning Ironman.

Then Allen hired coach Phil Maffetone, who had him do several months of easy aerobic training at the start of the season, followed by six weeks of very hard work. Allen won the Ironman six times.

Tim Noakes, author of *Lore of Running*, asked Allen why more triathletes hadn't adopted the methods that brought him so much success. "Allen answered that many athletes are too ego-driven. They can't wait to perform well and will not accept anyone else's ideas."[34]

Bill Aris's methods aren't what coaches want to hear. And that's too bad, because there's solid scientific evidence that the heart can work harder, with less strain, in the presence of happy feelings.

Coaches who support their runners, intent on helping

---

33. "Stotan: The Secret of Fayetteville Manlius," XCNation/RunnerSpace, September 23, 2013. http://www.runnerspace.com/news.php?news_id=180217

34. *Lore of Running*, op. cit.

them become happy contributors to a happy team, aren't wasting their time. They're creating a powerful training effect. They're making their runners better—by tapping the power of positive feelings to make each runner's heart a champion.

(As of this writing, in February, 2015, Bill Aris had begun work on a book about his experiences and his methods over the last 10 years.)

27. PLANNING MY NEXT LIFE AS A HIGH SCHOOL ATHLETE

I suspect I'm not the only washed-up old crock who dreams of being reborn and having another chance to play high school sports.

My high school experience in this life wasn't exactly distinguished or happy. I'm hoping that with careful planning, I can improve on it next time.

As a freshman, I ran track for a coach who spent no time—not a hundredth of a second—giving us instructions on technique, or explaining training, or making the slightest effort to motivate us.

I played football for the same coach. As a 14-year-old, 140-lb starter on the JV team, I scrimmaged daily with the varsity—they were short of linemen and used me to fill a hole, a function I didn't fill terribly well.

I vividly remember the practices where I faced varsity tackle Rex Mirich. One moment I would see Rex in front of me, and then the quarterback and I would find ourselves on our backs looking up at the sky, totally mystified about how it happened. Rex would play for the Raiders, Patriots, and Broncos.

When I return to this planet, what sport will I play? What kind of coach do I want to play for? How will I train? What attitudes will I bring to sports?

These are the kinds of questions I ask.

A major part of my reason for writing *The Joyful Athlete* was to answer those questions. I wrote the book, in part, so that I can start my next life with positive ideas about sports firmly implanted in my brain.

I want to be prepared to get more out of sports when I come back next time. How can I make it a more thrilling, challenging, high-energy, happy experience?

When I return, I hope the high school library will have a copy of *The Joyful Athlete*, so I'll be able to get a jump start on the answers.

Meanwhile, I'm trying to use my dwindling time wisely.

I spend hours cruising the Internet to learn about inspiring coaches and their methods.

I love to ponder the kinds of sports experiences that yield the greatest success and joy for young athletes.

Just yesterday, I ran across an incredibly interesting article by Tony Holler, "10 Reasons to Join the Track Team."[35]

Tony coaches track and field and freshman football at Plainfield North High School in Illinois, on the outskirts of Chicago, where he also teaches honors chemistry.

In 34 years as a coach, he's had eight individual state track champions and seven state champion relay teams. Which is NTS—not too shabby.

What makes me eager to run for Coach Holler (or more likely his grandson) when I'm reborn is the way he thinks about sports.

> My track program does not solely focus on the varsity level. We value freshmen and sophomores as much as we value juniors and seniors. . . .

---

35. "10 Reasons to Join the Track Team," http://www.freelapusa.com/10-reasons-to-join-the-track-team/

Do we minimize freshmen academically while we glorify seniors? Maybe I'm old school, but athletics should be a *classroom*, not a revenue-driven exercise in greed. Every kid should have a good experience, not just the gifted.

When I ran track as a high school freshman, our coach was a former college football lineman who spent all his time in practices hanging out with the big guys—the junior and senior weights men. They got a hundred percent of his attention.

I'll admit I was a poor runner. Our family had recently moved to Arizona from a mining camp at 7000' altitude in the Chilean Andes, where our main sports were skiing and hiking the high mountain valleys behind the town.

When it came to track, I didn't have a clue—I couldn't imagine what happiness a kid could possibly get out of running, or why I should take it seriously for any reason at all.

I ran because I thought my dad would be proud of me if I played football (*really bad idea*). And I'd heard that the football players were expected to come out for track to get fit for the coming season.

When Coach wasn't looking, my buddy Bruce and I would walk around the track, wisecracking. As a result, when Coach entered us in a mile race at a large high school in Tucson, I found myself increasingly far behind the rest of the runners.

Bruce did pretty well. When I dropped, he was 300 yards ahead of me. Bruce knew what he was doing. He regularly rode his bike or ran and walked 10 miles to school over hilly desert roads.

On one lap, I heard my embarrassed coach sheepishly tell another coach, "Well, I just have them run track to get them fit for football." As a result of my non-training, I was ill-prepared and dropped out. Coach screamed at me in front of the crowd, "You're the first person to quit at San Manuel High School!"

This is why, when I hear Tony Holler talk about actually *teaching* freshmen athletes, I get a little emotional.

Over the years, when I've finished a marathon or a 50-miler in a state of great grace and joy, I have sometimes turned inward and sent a cheery message into the distant past: "How about them apples, Coach?"

When I come back to this planet (or some other), what sport will I play? Probably not football. But it will be a team sport, where there will be a potential for camaraderie, and where young people can develop qualities like loyalty, respect, inner toughness, and where they can learn the joy of sacrificing their egos to achieve mutual goals.

I'll probably run cross-country. If I'm reborn with a very different body and mentality, I'd love to play water polo. And I'll surely run track. Tony Holler:

Unlike the ball-sports, track teams are not breeding grounds for jealousy and pettiness. Your spot on the team will be based on measured performance, not based on the opinion of your coach. Every kid that's ever sat the bench in a ball-sport has secretly hoped that a teammate would screw up. In track, we cheer for everyone, even our opponents. Track is not a zero-sum game. Your success is not based on your opponent's failure.

But here's the biggest reason I'll look for a coach like Tony:

"We need to keep our athletes happy. Happy athletes are the best recruiters."

Holler's ideas seem to mirror the coaching philosophy of Bill Aris, whose boys' and girls' teams swept the 2014 Nike

Cross Nationals (discussed in the last chapter), and Mike Scannell, coach of Grant Fisher, who won the Footlocker individual cross-country national championships in 2013 and 2014.

Both coaches are focused on efficient training that aims to help each athlete improve at his or her level.

That's the kind of coach I'd like to run for—someone who helps his athletes understand what they can get out of the sport, and how they can get there, starting where they are.

It works brilliantly. Over the years, Aris has had few superstar athletes on his teams. His genius is helping moderately talented kids realize their potential. At the 2014 NXN, the runners on his winning Fayetteville-Manlius boys' team placed 8, 14, 15, 19, 55. The winning F-M girls placed 11, 12, 13, 14, 20.

Under Mike Scannell's guidance, Grant Fisher ran just 50 miles a week and did *no speedwork*, while preparing to run a 4:02.3 mile and win Footlocker twice.

Scannell's focus, like Aris's, is on finding out what's best for the individual runner—Scannell says his goal is to send his runners home after each practice smiling, and never, ever burned-out.[36]

A current coaching dogma is that high school football players shouldn't play other sports. But in an article with the intriguing title "13 Things That Confuse Slow People," Holler draws on data from elite Division I football programs including Alabama, Auburn, and Baylor to show that the major predictors of a high school athlete's success in college and the NFL aren't size and raw strength, but speed and

---

36. "Smartest Training Ever of a High School Runner? Thoughts on Grant Fisher and Mike Scannell," http://www.joyfulathlete.com/2015/01/09/smartest-training-ever-high-school-runner-thoughts-grant-fisher-mike-scannell/

athleticism.

That's why he believes football players should run track, and why they should ignore coaches and athletic directors who try to get them to specialize.

We hear the same tired anti-cross-training propaganda in distance running: to become a better runner, you must focus on running. An essential principle of joyful sports is that success and happiness come when we *do what works*, not when we stay glued to untested but logical-sounding theories.

In recent years, we've seen a surprising number of elite high school distance runners who've been multi-sport athletes.

- Age-group champion triathlete **Lukas Verzbicas** ran a sub-4:00 mile while in high school.
- **Jordan Hasay** swam competitively until her high school junior year.
- **Allie Ostrander**, who won the 2014 Nike Cross Nationals and made it look easy, is a four-sport athlete in track, cross country, basketball, and soccer.
- **Grant Fisher**, the current top high school distance runner in the U.S., played soccer until his senior year.
- **Alexa Efraimson**, who won 1500m bronze at the 2013 IAAF World Youth Games, does long sets of hurdle mobility drills, medicine ball work, and calisthenics to build overall athleticism and explosiveness.
- **Katie Rainsberger**, sixth-place finisher at NXN in 2013, is a year-round runner and soccer player. Katie's mother, Lisa, the last American woman to win the Boston marathon (1984), says, "You don't have to be linear to be great. You don't have to focus only on running. You have to become an athlete. The progress in running will come from that."
- **Elise Cranny**, now at Stanford, was the number-

one high school distance recruit in the U.S. Cranny played soccer in high school.

- **Briana Gess** won the New Jersey state high school cross country championships as a 15-year-old freshman. Briana plays basketball. The runner-up was Josette Norris, a basketball player who ran a 4:41 1600m as a junior.
- 1984 Olympic marathon champion **Joan Benoit Samuelson** grew up as a skier.

Playing a second sport can give young runners a tremendous advantage.

- Cycling builds the main running muscles, the quads, without stressing the rest of the body.
- Swimming builds aerobic power without the stress of weight-bearing exercise.

As a result, a runner can train more, with shorter recovery.

When I come back next time, I guess I'll be a triathlete who runs track and cross-country.

If two sports are good—why not five?

28. FACEPLANT

Casting my mind over the faceplants of decades past, I find that each one has been rich with meaning.

I'll never be persuaded that faceplants occur randomly. I believe that they're formulated with apothecaric precision to cure us of our egotism.

(Early 1990s.) I'm running on a sidewalk in Sacramento during the early morning rush hour, with hundreds of cars whizzing by. I've lost weight and I'm in great shape, with a nut-brown tan. Naturally, this prompts my Inner Idiot to spread his feathers and caw: "I guess I'm showing these commuters what a really fit older runner looks like . . ." Bam splat. My bent little finger serves as a permanent reminder of the fruits of fatheadedness.

(Early 2000s.) I'm feeling frustrated—I don't remember why—and I unwisely decide to unload on God. I pray, none too humbly, "I can't figure out why the hell I'm having such trouble with this godda . . ." Bam splat.

Fifteen minutes later, I round a corner in the trail and the frustrations take hold again. I get no further than, "Goddamn it . . ." Bam splat. As I pick myself up, I don't know whether to laugh or cry. I think, "Maybe I'll share my frustrations with God in future, but I doubt I'll risk yelling at Him." At that point, I relax and become absorbed in humble appreciation of the beautiful day, and have a fine run.

(Early 1990s.) I'm tooling down a trail above the Yuba River during the Gold Country Marathon, a tiny race with just twelve entrants. The scenery is lovely—thick conifer and oak forest with fleeting views of the river. I'm trim, fit, and feeling not too bad about having passed someone who feels competitive with me. In short, I'm feeling complacently self-satisfied and happy to *be me* . . . Bam splat.

(Mountain View, California. 1996.) I've moved here to work with a legal team defending a lawsuit with important First Amendment implications. A jealous spiritual organization has sued our church, claiming it owns all rights to our teacher's books, pictures, and recordings. (It took 12 years, but we won 95% of the issues in the case. US law doesn't encourage religious monopolies.)

The day after I arrive, I'm running in the Palo Alto Baylands and thinking how great it is to be back in the Bay Area. I'm planning how I'll increase my mileage, enter local races, explore the trails of the Coastal Range, and . . . Bam splat.

At that point, I've had five sprained ankles in six weeks. This one is a rip-snorter—the ankle swells to grapefruit size; an X-ray reveals a hairline fracture.

The faceplant helps me get straight on my priorities. In my two years with the legal crew, I'm able to run regularly, but it's clear that running takes second place to our fight for religious freedom.

(Yesterday.) I've introduced three new training methods to my running, and it isn't working. It's too much. The details don't matter. But a clear intuition tells me to limit my weekly sub-threshold run to 25 minutes. However, I'm feeling so good that I try to jolly my intuition into letting me sneak in "just another 5, 10, 15 minutes" . . . Bam splat—worst faceplant in 40 years.

I slam hard into the gravel road. My hands and knees are bleeding, my breath is knocked out, and my nervous system and spine feel deeply battered. I rise with pain and limp to the finish. I spend the rest of the day and the next morning in a kind of bewildered shock.

Why? That's the question. The answer is surely that I've been using energy for running that I should have been applying to other things.

In an interview in *Running Times*, marathoner Ryan Hall reflected on the role his Christian faith plays in his training. The interviewer's unvoiced question was: "If you have so much faith in God, and if you spend so much time praying, how come you haven't won Boston, New York, London, and the Olympics?"

I'm no Ryan Hall. I don't lay it on the line against the Ethiopian and Kenyan elites who come to the marathon with 20,000 miles in their legs. But I'm almost three times as old as Ryan, and I've realized that God doesn't care if we win or lose. He cares about the lessons we learn along the way. Outward results matter a lot less than inner transformation.

Whether you view God as personal, or as an infinite intelligence and energy, or if you don't believe in God at all, it's clear that the lessons we learn from running have a definite direction.

It's as simple as this: the tough lessons teach us to do the right thing. We learn to heed the lessons because we suffer if we don't.

My faceplants happen when I go off course—when I harbor contractive thoughts and feelings. They aren't meant to hurt me, but to prevent me from hurting myself.

29. PICKIN' UP GOOD VIBRATIONS

Emerging from the Gare du Nord in Paris, I was delighted; not just to be seeing Paris for the first time, but by how the women dressed.

Walking to our hotel, not a block passed that we didn't see a creative statement, a one-off design that expressed the wearer's mood, taste, and aspirations. There was a vibration in the air of "Liberté, Egalité, Fraternité." The atmosphere breathed of creativity and freedom.

If you've visited Hawaii, you know that the air is like a massage. People return from the Islands looking as if they'd been pummeled by brown Lomi Lomi hands, faces flushed, eyes dreamy, skin radiating Aloha. Landing at SFO, the feeling is instantly colder—it's iced with Silicon Valley efficiency.

There's a northern California race, which for gentlemanly reasons I won't name, where the atmosphere is a killer.

Fifteen miles into the race, you feel as if your legs were melting into the pavement. It's a notorious black hole—a Bermuda Triangle that eats runners, laughs at their PR dreams, and emits evil anti-runner ions.

The weird thing is, the surroundings are beautiful. The course passes through lush farmland, punctuated by oak groves and meandering streams.

I've noticed similar anomalies on the routes I run nearer home. Some have wonderful energy. Others are energy sumps. Those courses make me want to lie down by the road and weep.

The worst routes are those where the first miles raise my hopes with positive vibes, only to dash them as the course traverses a Slough of Despond.

A route I no longer run is that way. It's on the Stanford campus.

I feel fine as I set out from the sports complex and jog past the Quad, the hospital, the community garden, the stables, the driving range, and the lake. I continue to enjoy the route, unmolested by any Furies beneath the road, as I jog the four-mile loop through the Stanford Hills, then descend to Stanford Avenue.

But I've learned to avoid Escondido Road. I mean—forget it. Perhaps it's the freshman dorms that line the street, oozing a hundred years of exam-book angst, a century-long drip of black bummer-oil that leaks from the pavement.

Perhaps it's my own melancholy freshman memories. The point is, bad vibes are something to watch out for.

I've been a runner long enough to notice that the trends of a runner's career have vibrations, too.

Forgive me if I revisit my memories of the Seventies. Back then, road races offered a colorful variety of mongrel distances. In the Bay Area, we had the 17-mile Berkeley-to-Moraga race, a point-to-point event that climbed the eucalyptus-lined Berkeley Hills, and descended into the burbs of the nation's 79th-wealthiest city. Another beautiful course followed the famed Seventeen-Mile Drive on the Monterey Peninsula.

Race directors 40 years ago weren't concerned with carefully measured distances. The standard 5K, 10K, half-marathon, 30K, and marathon events hadn't supplanted the

RDs' fertile imaginations. If they liked, they could string a course 15 miles between two random East Bay cities—say, Pleasanton to Livermore—just for the hell of it, and because they could.

Those races were fun. They were travelogues, adventures in places you'd otherwise never dream of running. By contrast, today's tidy 5K/10K loop courses seem sterile and uninspired, each like all the others. Pay your $40, run 20 minutes or an hour, grab a shirt, and there you go. Little races made of ticky-tacky.

Gosh, I'm sounding like a crabby old man. What an ugly face I have right now. It obvious why the standard distances have prevailed—it's a lot easier to set up a 5K than a meandering 17-miler. And standard distances allow us to compare results without hauling out a calculator.

Nevertheless, in too many areas of our lives there's been a trend toward conformity, efficiency—and boringness.

When populist running was suckling, in the late Sixties and early Seventies, it had an individualistic, counterculture feel. Frank Shorter had long hair and a moustache; as did Pre. Both spoke out against running's old-fogey establishment, those gray eminences of the AAU who defended a phony amateurism.

The spirit of the Seventies invited us to run as healthy hippies; only less whiny. Our feelings for the sport were captured by Wes Holman, the counterculture hero played by Bruce Dern in *On the Edge*, and Peter Strauss in *The Jericho Mile*. ("Without me coaching you, without Captain Midnight filling your hoochy soul with funky inspiration, how are you going to be champion?")

Dialing back in time to 1962, we had Tom Courtenay in *The Loneliness of the Long Distance Runner*. Those movies were about individualism against conformism, individual dreams versus The Machine.

I mentioned in an earlier chapter how I drove *Pepito*, my funky 1980 Honda Civic, to a race in Stockton, California, in 1990. Pulling into the parking lot, I spied a running buddy and ambled over. Carl was one of the world's nicest guys. A retired professor who'd taught at a university in Japan, he was listening to an older gentleman who looked as if he hadn't had a satisfactory bowel movement since 1948.

I climbed out of the car and strolled over, smiling at Carl while the old man impaled me with a frown, then turned and gazed balefully at my car, looking like a pterodactyl with a secret sorrow.

I thought, "He's one of the guys who are ruining running— the bean counters who weigh everything in dollars and status." I'd noticed his brethren since my return to running in 1988, after an eight-year hiatus due to illness. They were a new demographic of folks who were happiest while droning about their stock portfolios during group runs.

In 1997, Dave Littlehales and I ran the What, Mi-Wok? Trail 100K together. Actually, we power-walked it. A former 2:50 marathoner, Dave has congenital hip problems that prevent him from running.

Late in the race, a pair of trail sweeps trailed behind us, yakking loudly about the criminal cases they'd defended. Although we were fifty miles into the race, Dave and I sped up to get out of earshot.

Preemptive Disclaimer: I'm sure there's an attorney who's a really great guy, somewhere in the wilds of northern Minnesota. But, let's face it, if you run with lawyers and bean counters, you take your chances.

Does running need unspoken codes of behavior and

status? Resolved, that running should be about making good vibrations. Corollary: that the sport exists for the individual, regardless of religion, ethnicity, or bank balance.

I've mentioned *The Holy Science*, a little book published in 1894 by Sri Yukteswar, a master of yoga in Bengal. He wrote:

> When ... love, the heavenly gift of nature appears in the heart, it removes all exciting causes from the system and cools it down to a perfectly normal state, and envigorating the vital powers excretes all foreign matters—the germs of diseases—from it by natural way ... and thereby makes man perfectly healthy, in body and mind, and enables him to understand the proper guidance of nature.... Hence the culture of this love the heavenly gift is the principal thing for the attainment of holy salvation and it is beyond doubt impossible for man to advance a step towards the same without this.[37]

He listed eight "obstacles" that prevent us from making our hearts expansive. He called them "the meanness of the human heart": hatred, shame, fear, grief, condemnation, race distinction, pedigree, and sense of respectability.

Running delivers the richest rewards when we open our hearts—and when we steer clear of people and places that close them.

Happily, there are any number of ways to avoid the heart-narrowing trends in the sport and harvest good vibes. Running will always offer the escape of solo running, or running in nature with like-minded friends. In simple harmony with nature, our bodies relax, our minds clear, and our hearts soar free.

---

37. *The Holy Science*, op cit.

30. EVERY RUNNER'S FRIEND

When I stopped running ultras, I mentioned the fact to Joe Henderson.

Joe told me he'd noticed that a runner's career typically progresses in six- or seven-year stages. As an example, he recalled running his best marathons during a six-year period.

The notion that a runner's career advances in orderly, stepwise fashion fascinates me. Taking my cue from ancient wisdom, I believe that runners experience those stages in a specific order, which I described in chapter 3, "The Five Dimensions of Fitness."

The first six years are for the body. The focus at the start is on achieving basic fitness and answering body-related questions such as which shoes to wear, which fuels to take, how much to drink, how to increase mileage, how to train, how to carry water, etc.

Things get more interesting after we've answered those ground-level questions. In the second stage, we seek new adventures. We'll try a 10K, a half-marathon, maybe a full 26.2, or wow, an ultra. It's the "feeling stage," when a quest for inspiration fuels our running.

I smile when I remember how much I enjoyed the feeling phase. I ran in the Sierra foothills, always alone, padding through old-oak forests on narrow single-track trails with fragrant kitkidizze brushing my ankles.

It was during the feeling stage that I started collecting names for my imaginary yearly "Every Runner's Friend" award.

In December, my thoughts would turn to the runners who had inspired me in the last year—not just for their running but their human qualities.

I never write down the list; I carry it in my heart. It's a gathering of runners that I'm pretty sure I could talk to as friends, despite their elite status.

High on the list is Joe Henderson. Joe *is* every runner's friend—always has been, since I met him in 1970.

Another high-ranking runner is Mark Plaatjes. A former world marathon champion, Mark won his ERF award for two acts of friendship. First, for the sincere regret he felt at beating a friend in the World Championships marathon. Second, when injury forced him to drop out of the New York City marathon while he was running in the lead pack. Instead of whining, Plaatjes hobbled to the nearest first-aid tent, where he applied his skills as a professional sports therapist to massage the slower runners.

Then there's Ann Trason, the great ultrarunner. I'm aware that in *Born to Run*, Christopher McDougall flayed Trason for losing her cool at the Leadville Trail 100, the year she was in an all-out race against the male Tarahumara runners (and nearly beat them).

At one point, Trason glared at the *indios* while they refueled in the aid tent. McDougall seized on this to set Trason up as the prototypical über-competitive American who lost to the gentle, playful Tarahumara.

Nothing could be further from the truth. Trason was an elite runner in a branch of the sport that drew no prize money, no great fame, and no hype. She could have had a lucrative career as a road marathoner, but chose instead to run trail ultras because she loved the sport and the people.

Over the years, Ann inspired and helped many. At a 100-mile road race at Gibson Ranch in Sacramento, I watched as Trason, who wasn't entered, lovingly encouraged the leaders, running alongside Kevin Setnes and handing him fluids and wiping him down with a sponge.

I was delighted, both years I ran the Quad Dipsea, to find Ann working the aid station at Stinson Beach, handing out goodies for no reward other than the pleasure of helping old geezers like me. When I ran the What, Mi-Wok? Trail 100K, there was Ann, cheering the runners as they trundled through Tennessee Valley.

I've decided to retire Ann Trason's singlet—she'll be on my Every Runner's Friend list forever.

It's mid-January, but the voting hasn't closed. This morning I was happy to add a uniquely deserving runner to my list. After watching videos of talks by Dr. Armando Siqueiros, MD, a family physician in San Luis Obispo, California, I knew that if anyone deserved the Every Runner's Friend award, it was he.

What makes Dr. Siqueiros special is that he coached Jordan Hasay during her high school years. He did a better job than her coaches at the University of Oregon, in my opinion. But that's another story.

If you haven't heard of Jordan, you must be living in Uzbekistan. Hasay was the nation's most successful prep runner. She won the Footlocker Cross-Country Championships as a 14-year-old freshman, and again in her senior year.

I've added Dr. Siqueiros to my list for the wonderful way he managed Jordan's training.

Dr. Siqueiros had only been coaching two years when he met Hasay. He'd taken the coaching job as a volunteer when several boys at Mission Valley Prep decided they wanted to start a track team and requested his help.

With two years' experience and no credibility, he was handed the most sensationally gifted runner of her generation.

In several workshop videos, he talks about the difficulty of his situation—how everyone expected Jordan to set a course record each time she ran, if not a national record, and how the media hyped her endlessly.

The videos are informal, and Siqueiros's style is humble, thoughtful, and unpretentious. But as you listen, you begin to realize that his words carry deep wisdom.

As Hasay's coach, Siqueiros faced two obstacles. First, he was committed to ideas that went radically against how most coaches would have guided her training.

Second, he refused to use Hasay to satisfy the public's lust for sensation, or to promote his own reputation. From the start, he stood uncompromisingly at the gifted young runner's side, treating her as a valued individual.

At his initial meeting with Jordan and her parents, Dr. Siqueiros handed them a list of former Footlocker national champions, going back to the first Footlocker race. He asked them to look over the list and read the names of the Footlocker winners who had won an Olympic medal.

Silence.

He then asked them to name the Footlocker winners who had made the US Olympic team.

Silence.

Finally, he asked them to identify any Footlocker winners who had won an NCAA championship in college.

Silence. (Siqueiros later identified two or three runners

who'd won an NCAA title.)

He explained that he wasn't interested in exploiting Hasay's talent, and that chasing honors was much less important than her development as a runner who would have a long and enjoyable career. He promised to teach her how to train, how to plan her schedule, how to stay fresh, and how to avoid the burnout that had killed the careers of so many Footlocker champions.

Siqueiros soon had a chance to back up his words. Hasay had been invited to the prestigious Stanford Invitational cross-country meet, and Jordan and the family were excited about the trip. But Siqueiros told them she should decline the invitation, because she wasn't ready.

Hasay's parents were horrified. They ignored his advice and traveled to Palo Alto with their superstar daughter—who bombed badly and dropped out of the race.

Siqueiros' apparent ability to predict the future bolstered his credibility. In fact, his judgment was based on sound observation.

Hasay had shown amazing resilience in her training. She was never sore and never tired, no matter how hard or far she ran. The training she had designed for herself was simple: she ran six miles every day, as hard as possible, in an all-out race to beat her previous PR. When she succeeded, she was elated, and when she failed she was crushed.

In races against other high school teams, she went out hard, building a 30- or 40-yard lead in the first 100 yards. Siqueiros knew that at Stanford, running as a freshman against the best juniors and seniors from all over the West, this tactic would be a disaster. The other runners would bide their time, run their own race, and devour her in the stretch.

Siqueiros had won the Hasay family's attention. He set out

to teach Jordan a set of principles that echoed those espoused by Arthur Lydiard and Bill Bowerman.

He made mistakes, but in time he convinced her to stop racing in training, and he persuaded her of the wisdom of getting enough rest. He helped her stop obsessing over times, to forget the stopwatch and run by inner feeling. And he unfailingly placed her needs above the ambitions others held for her. He flatly ignored the expectations of other coaches and the national media, who continued to hype Jordan as a future college superstar and Olympian.

In fact, Siqueiros didn't "coach" Jordan Hasay. He guided and taught her. He saw her as a person, not a running machine designed to satisfy his and others' lust for glory. He simply didn't have those desires.

Siqueiros had a defining quality of great teachers: he put the student's needs first. He looked beyond short-term success and managed Jordan's training for the long haul. He was more concerned that she be healthy and happy, than that she win races and set records. As a result, Hasay looked as fresh and enthusiastic in her final Footlocker race as she had four years earlier.

Arthur Lydiard believed that America's high schools and colleges are perfectly designed to destroy the careers of runners. The hectic schedules, the doubling at meets, the two or three tough competitive seasons in nine months, tempt coaches to try to squeeze results from their runners by the most expedient means. They grab at training methods that improve a runner's speed in the short term, but contribute little or nothing to their long-term aerobic development.

Fortunately, that's beginning to change, as coaches like Dr. Siqueiros demonstrate that the best results come by taking a long view, and by focusing on the needs of the individual runner. It's the same view that Lydiard and Bowerman took with their elite runners.

Dr. Siqueiros, you're on the Every Runner's Friend List. Thank you for your inspiring example.

31. LET'S GET IT WRONG

What if we never made a mistake in our training?

What if we never overtrained. Never found ourselves on a long run, miles from anywhere, struggling in painful limp-home mode. Never took a wrong turn, never ate the wrong foods, never consumed too little fluids, never went out too fast. Wouldn't that be cool?

Hmm, maybe.

While taking precautions is good, being too careful can deprive us of valuable lessons. We can learn a lot by going out to the edge.

One of my favorite blogs, Marc McGuiness's *Lateral Action*, offers advice on creativity for artists, writers, and business people. (www.lateralaction.com)

In a post, "Fear of Getting It Wrong," Mark offered six suggestions that artists can follow to stay "fearlessly creative."

Here's how I interpret them for runners:

1. Write with Your Body. Is there a runner who hasn't come home bursting with creative ideas? Those ideas come when we turn off the nitpicking mind, enjoy the flow of pure energy, and open ourselves to receive them.

2. Stop Worrying. When the micro-managing mind takes over, it's harder to listen to the body's whispered wisdom.

3. Start Getting Things Wrong. We can often get a fresh perspective by going out on a limb. Try blasting through a planned easy run. Add some hard tempo at the end of your 2½-hour run. Try doing 30-mile run/walks with *no fuels at all*, just water and electrolytes. I've made these mistakes—and learned priceless lessons.

4. Stick Two Fingers Up at the Critics. New runners often accept others' ideas uncritically. But *no one can tell you how to train.* The best coaches know this. Arthur Lydiard and Bill Bowerman preached *principles.* They rarely gave detailed advice. They knew that, as Lydiard put it, "a runner's conditions change" and their training needs to be adjusted every day.

5. Get Good Feedback. If you don't have a coach or mentor, you can get excellent feedback from books, especially those penned by the sport's wise elders. For my money, our wise teachers are legends like Lydiard and Bowerman. My favorite book on training is Keith Livingstone's comprehensive Lydiard guide, *Healthy Intelligent Training.*

6. Grant Yourself Poetic License. McGuinness quotes poet e.e. cummings:

and even if it's sunday may i be wrong
for whenever men are right they are not young

Give yourself poetic license to scrap your plan and do what's most appropriate on the day. If you do the right thing—slow down, go home early, run harder—you might find that your body responds gratefully and rewards you with unexpected joy.

Training isn't linear. It isn't a point-to-point race on a seamless asphalt highway. It's a gnarly, twisting forest trail. It's good to keep an eye on the ground and react appropriately.

"The perfect is the enemy of the good." I find this simple principle applies equally well in my work as a writer and runner, not to mention my "career" as a (very) amateur singer, and my 48-year meditation practice.

Seymour Papert is a professor of computer science at MIT. Papert co-invented the LOGO programming language for children. He believes that one of the most valuable lessons kids learn from programming is a "debugging approach to life."

Professional programmers make as many as 100 mistakes per 1000 lines of code they write. The mistakes are an accepted part of the process. Papert believes life is like that—it's silly to fear that we won't get it right the first time. Better to plunge ahead with enthusiasm and fix things as we go.

As a writer, I'm comfortable pouring crap into a first draft. I'm not discouraged when the initial effort reads like garbage, because I know that, buried in that awful muck, is the germ of an idea that will shine forth when I shovel away the mound of ordure under which it's hiding.

In the early 1970s, I edited a magazine for bicyclists. I told new writers not to worry about the quality of their writing. I told them we didn't care if they scrawled their articles in crayon on a brown-paper bag, so long as they had good *ideas*.

As a meditator, I've learned how hard it is to persuade the mind to slow down and focus. I discovered early on that I could speed the process if I didn't work with the mind, but if I tried to find the place in my heart where I could rest with positive, harmonious feelings.

When we love something, the mind loves to concentrate on it.

I recall one meditation vividly. I had done something that I wasn't entirely proud of. In meditation that evening, I said, "Well, I guess You'll just have to accept me as I am." I was surprised to hear a brisk motherly voice that said: "I am not concerned with your faults. I am concerned only with your *continual improvement."*

When I started running, I found that the "debugging approach" was the best way to go. It took thousands of miles to begin to understand what good training is like, how it feels, and how to do it consistently.

I made endless mistakes, including some howlers, but I gradually learned what felt right.

Mistakes are unavoidable. A good way to live with them is to be somewhat childlike. Build your sand castles without being too concerned about the result. Enjoy the process, then tear the castle down with a hearty laugh and start over, having found a better way.

32. INSIDE-OUT RUNNING

I'm reading Robert McKee's highly regarded book, *Story: Substance, Structure, Style, and the Principles of Screenwriting*. The book begins:

Story is about principles, not rules.

A rule says, "You must do it this way." A principle says, "This works ... and has through all remembered time." The difference is crucial.... Anxious, inexperienced writers obey rules. Rebellious, unschooled writers break rules. Artists master the form.

Lordy Bess, if that doesn't describe training, I just don't know! All of the joys of running, and all success, come by "mastering the form."

Inexperienced runners obey rules. At the start of my career, I read books and tried to apply the recommended schedules religiously. And I recall what an excruciatingly boring way it was to train, and how unsuccessful it was.

If the book said "Run 5 miles on Tuesday," that's what I did. And it wasn't long before I stopped obeying the "rules," because my body's needs were horribly ill-matched to those inflexible "systems."

I had equally poor results when I broke the rules. Running "however I felt" was a disaster. My emotions were a poor guide.

Years later, as I learned the *principles* of good training, and the value of calm feelings, I began to enjoy my running much more.

I found my way to the principles by two paths. Arthur Lydiard expressed them in crystal-clear outline. He taught his runners to tune every run to the needs of their individual bodies every day.

Lydiard taught important principles—periodization, the importance of the aerobic base, etc.—all based on his experience.

Robert McKee talks about the difference between writing screenplays "from the outside in," and from inside out.

Writers who start from the outside, says McKee, are rarely successful. They get a wonderful idea for a movie and then rush to start writing dialogue. It's a building-blocks approach: "I've got five great scenes—if I write great dialogue, I can hang the scenes together and create a great script!"

McKee's students have won 18 Oscars and 107 Emmys, so he knows what he's talking about, and he's seen his share of bad scripts.

What happens to writers who work "from the outside in"? If the script gets a reading at all, it's rejected with a remark such as "Very nicely written—good crisp, actable dialogue—vivid scene description, fine attention to detail, the story sucks. PASS ON IT."

And isn't that the trouble with planning our training "from the outside in"?

"I want to raise my VO$_2$Max and get faster at 5K and 10K. I'll do a ton of intervals and I'll get really good at interval running (scene A). But I also want to improve my endurance-at-speed for the half-marathon, so I'll do lots of tempo runs at 10K pace (scene B). With those excellent ingredients, my training can't fail!"

Those are great "scenes." But unless the plan works from start to finish—unless it tells a good story—it doesn't have a hope of a whisper of a micron of a chance of delivering the results we're after.

McKee describes the opposite process—"writing from the inside out." It takes months, as the writer scribbles ideas for scenes on 3x5 cards. As time passes, he subjects his ideas to ruthless scrutiny. In the end, perhaps none of the original cards remain. He works by principles. He knows how a great story feels, "and he won't be satisfied with anything less."

Okay, all analogies break down sooner or later—but there's a great deal about the inside-out process that mirrors good training.

Keep your attention on the long view. Be patient. Destroy everything that isn't good training. Be eternally on the lookout for quality. Know that you won't succeed unless you get the details right, and that each detail is only "right" when it accurately reflects valid principles. See the big picture—make sure every aspect of your training helps tell the story.

Training is an art. Like a great film, the end product can be satisfying, soulful, and beautiful. "A writer secure in his talent knows there's no limit to what he can create, and so he trashes everything less than his best on a quest for a gem-quality story."

33. MALE AND FEMALE AT THE RACES

I'm gazing at the results board after a 30K race in Sacramento, and I'm thinking dark thoughts.

Grinding my teeth, I grouse: *"There's no way that guy will beat me for third place in my age group if I do another month of speedwork."*

I linger near the board, grimly planning my training for the coming months.

A fit-looking woman in her thirties walks up and checks the board. Another woman approaches and says, "Oh—hi!!! I haven't seen you in such a long time! It's so good to see you! Which race did you run? How did you do?"

"Hi, it's great to see you, too! I ran the 30K. I placed third in my age group."

"That's *wonderful!!* I'm so happy for you! Congratulations!!"

The women chat and catch up on their lives.

I'm laughing inside. I'm thinking, "The universe is talking to me. Women know something guys don't. They've got their priorities in order."

It strikes me how cold it was to obsess over beating the other runner. I vow to train with joy, enjoying the process and letting the results fall where they may.

Running is male and female, a balance of feeling and reason, will power and relationships. Each has its role; both are needed; running without one or the other is incomplete.

34. NEXT GENERATION RUNNING

Why is *Star Trek: The Next Generation* so enduringly popular, its characters the most memorable of all the Trek series?

Surely it's because the construction of Next Generation mirrors life.

Geordi, Troi, Worf, Data, Picard. The five lead characters of *Next Generation* represent Body, Heart, Will, Mind, and Soul. These are, as I've repeated ad nauseam in this book, the five "tools" of a runner.

Running well requires that we run like Geordi, tending the source of our energy: our warp core, the body.

It demands that we run with Deanna Troi's intuition, swiftly piercing the truth of each situation, while bypassing the slow analytical grindings of the rational mind.

Good runs demand that we run with Worf's indomitable will, and Data's instant recall of the mechanical facts of training.

Finally, on those hopefully not-rare occasions when we manage to get all of the tools working in harmony, we'll find ourselves running as integrated beings, expressing health, love, strength, wisdom, and joy—like Jean-Luc Picard. Or Riker, the Master's apprentice.

Riding herd on the five tools of a runner isn't always easy; sometimes it feels like herding cats. A good way to get them all working together is by going straight to the heart.

When raw energy, logic, and force of will fail the Next Generation crew, they turn to Deanna Troi, whose wise, heart-born insights always prove correct.

Similarly, when we need answers for our training, tuning in to the heart's calm intuitions can usually save the day.

Run long and prosper. Oops! Wrong series.

35. SEASONS OF A RUNNER

Are all runners the same?

How different can we be? Don't we all train with arms, legs, a heart, and lungs?

Listen to David Costill, one of the world's most respected sports physiologists.

When I coached Bob Fitts (champion distance runner who is now one of the most prominent muscle researchers in the U.S.), we used to have heated arguments about performance. He would insist that anybody could be a champion if they trained hard enough. He's since changed his opinion. Now, he admits: "Oh no, it's genetics." If you start looking at genetics in a four-hour marathoner and a 2:05 guy, they are markedly different. (From an interview in *Runner's World Daily*.[38])

A *Newsweek* story, "Why Stress May Be Good for You,"[39] revealed just how closed-minded scientists can be. The author describes how mainline psychologists and physiologists have stubbornly rejected a large body of research which suggests that moderate stress is actually good for us:

In the short term, it (stress) can energize us, "revving

38. "Chat: Dave Costill," *Runner's World*. http://www.runnersworld.com/elite-runners/chat-dave-costill

39. Mary Carmichael, "Why Stress May Be Good for You," *Newsweek*, February 13, 2009.

up our systems to handle what we have to handle," says Judith Orloff, a psychiatrist at UCLA. . . .

When Orloff described her findings to other scientists, they basically told her that good stress doesn't exist.

A common belief is that adults who believe they thrive under stress may have been abused as children or exposed in the womb to high levels of adrenaline and cortisol.

Isn't that amazing? After reading the article, I thought, "Ask a marathoner or ultrarunner. They'll absolutely tell you that stress can be wonderful."

If running teaches us one thing, it's that the hardest races and workouts often produce the highest highs and the best memories.

The *Newsweek* article pointed out that the "inventor" of stress, endocrinologist Dr. Hans Selye, made a distinction between "bad" and "good" stress, which he called "eustress."

Stress develops concentration, emotional toughness, and will power: all essential tools of a runner. The stress of running—obviously, within limits—is like winter winds that strengthen a sturdy oak tree.

36. A RUNNER STUMBLES

Running teaches us that that it's a good idea to be gentle with our mistakes.

We can't avoid learning hard lessons—we're bound to get overtrained, injured, dehydrated, under-fueled, frozen and overheated—often for reasons that were nobody's fault but our own.

Great athletes learn to manage their mistakes. Consider tennis legend Pete Sampras. Watching Sampras play, his composure stood out. It was an important weapon in his arsenal—an uncanny ability to remain, or appear, unruffled after losing a point or committing a fault.

Sampras laid out his approach in his autobiography, *A Champion's Mind: Lessons from a Life in Tennis*, co-authored with Peter Bodo. It's a great read.

Watching Sampras late in his career, it was hard to imagine the young player who often stumbled. A quality that set him apart was his relaxed confidence. As he puts it in the book, he knew he would be successful; mistakes were just learning experiences.

Sampras was never a "head case." He was about acting and learning from his experiences. He didn't waste energy brooding over setbacks.

Athletes err when they assume that once they "get it right" they can relax. It's refreshing to learn that Sampras's confidence was based on repeating a single small aspect of a particular stroke hundreds of times in practice, until it became an automatic part of his play.

We can find enlightening words on practice in another inspiring biography, *The Genius—How Bill Walsh Reinvented Football and Created an NFL Dynasty*, by David Harris.

I've mentioned how, in Walsh's first year as coach of the San Francisco Forty Niners, the team was reeling, having suffered an abysmal 2-14 season. When Walsh took over, he set about rebuilding the team from the ground up, starting with practices:

> Bill abhorred wasted time on the practice field and thought it stupid to make his players prove how tough they were every day in practice. He wanted his players constantly busy improving themselves instead. He kept his practices short, but every minute was scripted and performed on a strict timetable, with players sprinting from one segment to the next. He emphasized practicing techniques with precision and attention to detail, over and over. He felt that skills often broke down late in games and that the only insurance against this was endless repetition, creating a muscle memory that freed players from thinking about what they were supposed to do and let them react automatically.

I can't resist repeating a story that Hall of Fame quarterback Joe Montana told at Walsh's funeral.

Montana threw an interception in an important game. When he returned to the bench, Walsh glared at him. Instead of looking away, his usual custom, Montana held the coach's eye. Walsh said, "What was that?"

Montana replied, "That was an interception." Walsh paused, then said with a faint smile, "And it was a darn good one. But let's not do it again."

A key to making each moment of training valuable is to be intensely *interested*. When our hearts are engaged in what we're doing—even if it's just jogging through an easy recovery run or a warmup—every moment can be enjoyable. If we pay attention and savor the moments, we're sure to find happiness and success.

37. SOLVING THE RIDDLE OF TRAINING

All hail the runner who knows how to train—who never doubts, questions, or wonders.

I've known runners like that. They seemed to know exactly what their bodies needed at all times. They were rarely overtrained. They didn't waste energy poring through books and articles. They just ran.

Carl Ellsworth was that kind of runner. On a quiet evening 20 years ago, Carl walked into the market where I worked. Seeing my Jedediah Smith Ultra t-shirt, he invited me to join a group that met once a week for speedwork at the local high school track.

I had done long, slow distance for years. I was ready for a change. Speedwork sounded perfect.

I showed up on Wednesday, eager to learn what Carl had to say.

Trouble is, he said nothing. Just, "Let's do three miles."

That was it. No explanation of the whys or wherefores. Just "Let's do three times 1 mile."

Each week, it was the same. In his quiet voice, Carl would announce the day's workout, always in a single sentence, and off we would go. We did our speedwork to the same, uncomplicated formula: three miles in combinations of quarters, halves, and miles, as hard as we could run. No heart monitors, or elaborate calculations based on "race pace."

We simply blasted off and went as fast as we could for the prescribed distance.

Come to think of it, Carl did explain his philosophy one evening. Again, he said it in a single sentence: "If you run hard in practice, it feels easy when you race."

Carl was 64. He had a gentlemanly demeanor and a wonderful runner's look, with snowy-white, shoulder-length hair, and a gnarly, weather-worn face. He'd been a professor of political science at a Japanese university. Now retired, his occupation, as far as I could tell, was full-time runner. He spent summers in the foothills of the Sierra and winters in Hawaii. His Japanese-born wife, Suru, spoke no English.

In Japan, there's an expression: *wabi-sabi*. It's a cultural and artistic movement based on appreciation for things gnarly, old, earthy, countrified, impermanent, and shaped by nature. Carl was *wabi-sabi*. Here's the Wikipedia's definition:

Wabi-sabi represents a comprehensive Japanese world view or aesthetic centered on the acceptance of transience. . . . Characteristics of the wabi-sabi aesthetic include asymmetry, asperity, simplicity, modesty, intimacy, and suggest a natural process.

That was Carl. He was simply himself.

When Carl's house burned down, several carpenter friends of mine helped him rebuild. They would tease Carl: "How come you're so *nice*, Carl? You're the *nicest* man we know!"

Carl and I met up with another runner in Sacramento for a final 20-mile tune-up before the California International Marathon.

Nearly every runner we passed greeted Carl with a smile. He *was* nice. He was likable because he was simple, modest, quiet, dignified, good-natured, and natural. People felt comfortable with him. Behind the gnarly exterior, there was

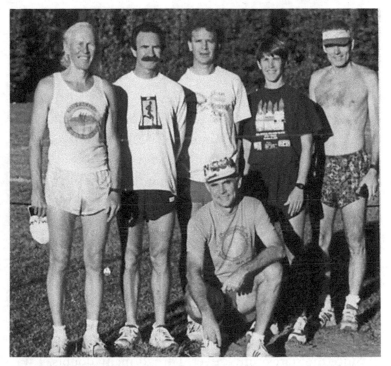

Carl Ellsworth, left, with the fast runners of the over-forty speedwork group at Nevada Union High School, 1995. Kneeling is Superior Court Judge John Darlington, member of a 4 x 1-mile team that set an age group world record. John ran a 4:05 mile in college despite asthma. At far right, in the nude, is the celebrated Swedish Olympian, Arnie Oldandslow.

a good heart.

Carl simply knew how to train. Or, rather, he had no doubts. My analytical mind found much to question about Carl's methods. For example, he never drank fluids during a marathon. Say *what!?* His explanation, characteristically simple, was: "I'm only out there three hours." But he had frequent gastric problems, and I'm guessing dehydration played a role.

Nevertheless, his style of training brought results. At 64,

he ran a 3:05 marathon. He'd run sub-3:00 many times, including the previous year. For three years straight, he won the northern California USATF road race series in the 60–65 age group.

His simple training worked for me. In my first session with the group, I struggled to run 3 x 1 mile with a best time around 7:35. After seven months of weekly "3 miles hard" I ran a 10-mile race in 70 minutes, at age 53.

Where did Carl's confidence come from? People who are filled with doubts are often defensive, loud, and blustery. But Carl was quietly assured. My guess is that he'd honed his self-assurance during the years when he ran 100-mile weeks and raced often. He appeared to have learned about running *by* running.

My own career was different. If I were to guess, I'd say that a higher power placed me in Carl's group so that I could learn the value of learning by doing, without over-thinking.

Since the start of my career, I'd had many doubts. I was fine for the first three years, when I simply ran at a high aerobic pace and kept trying to go a bit farther.

Then I took a job at *Runners' World,* and my training fell apart. Suddenly I was surrounded by runners who did things differently. They had complicated scientific explanations for their favorite blends of mileage, speedwork, long runs, heart rate, and pace. And they'd all been running 10, 20, 30 years. Who was I to question? I'd barely been running four years.

Where formerly I had run from my heart, intuitively, I was now overwhelmed by mental doubts. I felt there was a big Eye watching me, analyzing what I did, questioning and judging. "This book says ___, but this article says the opposite!" Surely there had to be a single, precise, *right* way to train. And if I wasn't doing that single, best, *correct* training, wasn't I just *wasting my time?*

It was like Zeno's paradox. At any instant, an arrow in flight isn't moving, because the instant is a snapshot in time. Therefore, if the arrow cannot move in a single instant, it cannot move in *any* instant. Therefore the arrow cannot move.

It's nutty-cakes, because it's using logic to break the fluid, uninterrupted motion of an arrow into small pieces. Zeno's paradox is intended to illustrate the limitations of logic and reason.

I made a similar mistake. I tried to break running into too many tiny parts.

I eventually realized that the times I "knew" with complete certainty how to train were when there was a strong feeling of rightness in my heart.

Carl Ellsworth was a scientist. He quietly tested his methods. And the "proof" was a 3:05 at age 64.

Carl was a polished runner. He was a work of art. In his *wabi-sabi* way, he was a beautiful man.

I've moved on since 1995. As I look back over my career, I realize I've learned the most by running and paying attention, while not thinking too much—like Carl.

Along the way, I've refined the instrument that lets me hear my body's lessons. That instrument is the calm, expansive heart.

Tuning my heart allows me to run hard, even as an old man. I still make mistakes. It's part of learning. But I'm no longer as confused as I was 36 years ago, when I worked at *Runner's World.*

38. SONG OF THE ROAD

An article in the *Independent* (UK) described research that showed listening to rock music extends a runner's endurance by as much as 15%.

Personally, I think the timing of the study couldn't be better, since it confirms my belief that in future music will be a standard tool of sports training.

While the evidence from the study isn't resoundingly convincing, and it a leaves a host of questions unanswered (1. Which music is best? 2 . . .), I suspect the findings will come as no surprise to the thousands of iPod-plugged-in Borg-Who-Run.

I use music continually while I run. I hum, sing inwardly, and sometimes feel so wonderful that I sing aloud. And I can't help but notice that it's possible to get a stronger, more lasting effect from *making* music than by listening passively.

During the California International Marathon, bands play along the route. I noticed that my energy would soar as we passed a band, whether it was the thump-thump of a high school marching band, the haunting chant of a bagpiper, or a rock band cranking out the usual strangle-juice. (Forgive me, I'm old. Most rock music sounds to me like beer cans being fed through a wood chipper.)

But I couldn't help but notice that my energy swiftly returned to its average level when I moved on.

Mark Allen, the legendary triathlete who won the Hawaii Ironman six times, is the author of an intriguing book, *Mark Allen's Total Triathlete*.

Allen urges athletes to "protect their power." He tells stories of triathletes who allowed themselves to be psyched-out by their competitors, and performed poorly as a result. The lesson he drew from those experiences is that we must be on our guard against lowering our necks in the presence of our competitors, lest they drop the axe.

While I believe there's no value at all in puppying-up to anyone, least of all some arrogant athlete, I wonder if Allen understood the amazing power of positive, expansive feelings.

I suspect that, like most people, he visualized anything but warriorly self-control as weak submission. In my view, the warrior's heart sustains and drives him. His heart isn't weakly sentimental; it's charged with a power that nothing and no one can withstand.

I can speak confidently about that power, because I've observed it in my spiritual teacher. I've seen him face hostile people with complete tranquility, without "giving up his power." He never fell into the error of brittle defensiveness.

I remember a day, about 30 years ago, when I visited his home for a private talk. When I arrived, a man from the neighborhood was sneeringly berating my teacher over some local political issue.

I fumed. I wanted to strangle the guy for the disrespectful way he was talking. But my teacher was completely calm, utterly relaxed and kindly. While not accepting the man's arguments, he treated him with utmost respect and compassion. After the man left, my teacher sighed and said, with complete sweetness, "Well, that ____ can be a pill."

A friend told me about a hot summer day when my teacher

was at a local lake, swimming with friends. A group of Hell's Angels roared up on their motorcycles. They dismounted and approached, making threatening remarks. My teacher silently stood but didn't say a word. The bikers turned on their heels and walked hastily back to their bikes, shouting, "We'll be back—we'll get you!" Of course, nothing happened. The ancient scriptures say that in the presence of a person who has perfected non-injury, no harm can arise.

I've felt the force of my spiritual teacher's love, which comes from his inner attunement with a bliss that is unbounded. It is not a sentiment; it is resoundingly powerful.

I believe the active heart is *it*, in sports and life. The passive heart never gets us anywhere.

I like to drive to San Francisco to run. I work in front of a computer screen all week, and I enjoy heading out of town to run across the Golden Gate Bridge and onto the beautiful trails of the Marin Headlands. It's an adventure run with wonderful views of sailboats on the Bay, an enormous cargo ship crossing under the bridge and tooting its horn, the international crowd promenading on the bridge walkway, and the amazing vistas of the Bay as the Coastal Trail ascends to the crest of the Headlands.

The main thing I get from the trip is the opportunity to sing during the drive to the City. I always notice that the better my singing goes, the better the run goes. When I'm able to put strong energy and feeling into my singing, it warms up and harmonizes my heart for the run. As I mentioned in chapter 5, scientists at Heartmath Institute have found that the heart's power output increases 500 to 600 percent in the presence of positive, expansive feelings such as love, kindness, compassion, etc., compared to passive "good feelings."

The Heartmath scientists discovered that the heart can

work much more efficiently when its beats are harmonized by those energizing expansive feelings. I find I can run fast with much greater ease when I expand my heart's feelings by singing for a long time in the car.

The Heartmath scientists have discovered a connection between calm, positive feelings and intuition. After singing my head off, I find I make better decisions, because I know in my heart what's right.

Nothing against iPods. But (apologies to the Beatles), listening passively just takes me half the way there. What happens when the iPod battery runs down? I say, mix it up, do a little singing, *con brio*, and turn your running into a whole new song.

39. STRANGE RAYS

Ian Jackson was an interesting guy. Back when dinosaurs still roamed the San Francisco Peninsula, we shared a run-down apartment on the wrong side of the tracks, a short walk from *Runner's World* where we shared an office. (Ian passed away in 2011.)

Ian was a talented athlete. He won the Pacific Division AAU (now USATF) 50K championship. In college, he trained with the UC Berkeley swim team.

Ian had an adventurous spirit. He had surfed big waves in Hawaii, had stowed away on an ocean liner bound for Australia (he was caught and returned), and had dived from 90-foot cliffs in Mexico.

Ian once ran 140 miles in the Berkeley hills while fasting for a week on plain water. During the final run, he experienced an expansion of consciousness, feeling that the eucalyptus trees swaying and creaking were part of his own greater being.

Ian used a phrase that bugged me. He would say, "Oh, (a person, book, idea) gives me energy." At first it seemed elitist—"If they *don't* give me energy, I won't have anything to do with them." But in time, I realized that he was right—upbeat people lift our spirits and give us energy. Life is too short to waste it on earth's Eeyores.

I got a phone call from Ian several years ago. We caught

up on the last 30 years and it was a delight. Ian was as full of beans as he'd been in 1975. He was living in Texas, where he advised runners and racing cyclists.

He told me about a breathing technique he'd discovered, that helps athletes crank up their energy. He described his work with the US Olympic cyclists at the national development center, where he shared his methods with Lance Armstrong's coach, Chris Carmichael. After the Olympics, Ian tried to stay in touch, but Carmichael didn't return his calls.

Fast-forward several years. Ian gets a call from a former French Tour rider who's now a journalist for a cycling magazine. He's familiar with Ian's Breathplay methods and is excited about something he witnessed during the previous season's Tour.

"I was in a press car and we were following the leaders on a long climb. I told the driver to pull up close to Lance, because I wanted to study his form. As we drew near, I could hear his breathing and I noticed that the rhythm was very unusual. Then it struck me: 'Oh my God, it's the same pattern as on the Breathplay CDs!'"

Ian sent me the CDs, and this morning I got a hint of their power. I ran two hours by the Bay, going slowly for an hour and 20 minutes, then did eight all-out 2-minute repeats.

At I started the repeats, I noticed I was breathing with the rhythm that Tim Noakes says most runners adopt while running: four steps on inhalation, four on exhalation while jogging; two steps in/out while running fast.

I was breathing in the 2:1 ratio—a breath for every two steps. But on the fourth or fifth repeat, my breath fell naturally into the rhythm that Ian had told me about: a quick inhalation followed by a much longer out-breath—in my case about four times as long.

What it did for my energy was amazing. The hard pace became easier and I was able to turn up the throttle, even though I'd been blasting along at 93% to 94% MHR.

After the run, my thoughts turned to other unusual experiences I've had with breathing.

You've probably experienced this. You're cruising along toward the end of a long run, finding a groove and feeling efficient, and you notice that you're barely breathing at all.

How can that be? It contradicts a basic axiom of physiology: the harder you run, the more oxygen you need, and the harder you must breathe.

I wonder if subtle energies are at play, energies that Western sports science knows nothing about.

I once hitched a ride with an interesting young man. He drove an old station wagon, had long hair, wore a necklace of large wooden beads, and sat very straight behind the wheel.

I asked him about the huge drum in the back of the car. He said, "It's part of my spiritual practice. I've studied tai ch'i for many years, and I've gotten past the physical part, to where I'm working with energy and sound—music and the voice."

He told me about a drum gig he'd played at a bar in Reno, where an all-hands fight broke out. "I projected my voice and the room instantly calmed down," he said. He told me he was returning to Reno to visit his teacher, because he needed to gain better control over the energy he'd awakened through the sound methods.

"I was attacked by a guy in the street. I didn't respond physically but sent energy out toward him," he said. "He ended up in the hospital with a serious heart rhythm disturbance. That's why I need to see my teacher."

At a Japanese cultural festival in the 1980s, I watched

a demonstration by an Aikido instructor. He was a burly Mexican-American man from San Jose. He held a simple wooden rod pointed forward, and his students ran full-tilt toward him, one by one.

He said, "I am projecting the power of love through the stick." Before a student reached the rod, he or she would slam back as if hitting an invisible wall. None of them were injured—they were all smiling.

Ray Krolewicz is a talented ultramarathoner who trains up to 200-plus miles a week. Ray has run many 2:37 marathons—on the way to running 100K (62.2 miles) in under 7 hours!

"RayK" once remarked that he only began to make real progress as a runner when he "learned to breathe"—a statement he unfortunately wouldn't elaborate on.

Former pro triathlete John Douillard is the author of an interesting book, *Body, Mind, and Sport*. Douillard advises athletes to breathe through their noses.

In one of our case studies on breath rate during a bicycle stress test, we found that as the exercise load increased, the breath rate went up, peaking for the subject . . . at 47 breaths per minute using conventional mouth breathing. At the maximum breath rate, all of our subjects were anaerobic, gasping for air and pushing right to the edge of their capacity.

The same subject was tested two days later on the same stress test, except that he used nasal breathing. This time the breathing was comfortable the entire time, even at the highest level of stress, and the average breath rate was 14 breaths per minute. This result is even more impressive when you consider that the average breath rate for people at rest is around 18 breaths per minute. (*Body, Mind, and*

Sport, 151–52)

I discovered Douillard's book when I was running ultramarathons. It took 2–3 weeks to get comfortable enough with nose-breathing that I could do it for seven hours during a 30-mile training outing. I did those runs slowly, so I can't report on the results at speed, but I did feel noticeably more relaxed, focused, and fresh while breathing through my nose.

Yoga recommends nose-breathing as a way to calm the mind. The reason given is that it energizes the brain's prefrontal cortex, where calm concentration is localized.

Douillard gives examples of athletes who struggled for several weeks with breathing through their noses, then found that they could run fast with a significantly slower heart and breath rate.

In *Lore of Running's* 900-plus pages, there are just two pages on the breath, but they're useful ones. Author Tim Noakes states that breathing with the diaphragm ("belly breathing") is more efficient than breathing with the chest muscles.

What he doesn't mention is that a straight posture makes abdominal breathing easier.

I can't cite research on this, but I'm convinced that a bent spine prevents the lungs from filling fully. I find that straightening my upper spine enables me to breathe easier at any pace. Most world-class marathoners run with straight backs, as if to make room for maximum lung expansion.

A remarkable feature of Frank Shorter's Olympic marathon victory in 1972 was his form. Shorter and his teammates at the Florida Track Club practiced running with their spines erect, with little forward lean and their center of gravity balanced directly over the pelvis. Shorter made sub-5:00 pace look easy—he appeared to be floating over the ground.

Yoga says there's a link between posture and energy. Language in every culture reflects this connection. When we feel negative, our spines bend and we say "I feel down," "I'm lower than a dachshund's belly," etc.

When our mood is positive, we say "I'm high." "I'm up." "I'm on top of the world."

Yoga lore says that negativity creates a downward movement of energy in the spine, making the spine feel weak and pliable. When we feel positive, there's an upward current that makes the spine feel strong and straight.

A useful practice from yoga that I enjoy is to deliberately breathe deeply during the warmup. I find it helps create a vortex of energy in the lungs, heart, and upper spine. I do this often, because it helps me feel centered in the heart and upper spine, a pleasant, positive feeling. I generally breathe in to a count of 8 or 12, then hold and exhale to the same count. The longer I practice, the more I feel pleasantly centered in the upper body.

Another helpful way to straighten the upper spine and neck is by bending backward, optionally clasping hands behind the back and stretching to "open the chest and make room for the heart."

These practices can make a big difference. Our posture is intimately linked to our worldview. Positive people tend to stand straight. Whiners slump. After doing the backbend and chest-stretch, you'll feel more like Frank Shorter, less like Joe Slob.

The heart is an important center of energy and consciousness. Running "from the chest and heart" is a wonderful feeling—it feels subtly right and liberating and generates confidence and power.

40. INTUITIVE RUNNER

Does intuition exist? Is it a reliable tool for a runner's training?

Research that I described in chapter 6 shows that it's easy to prove intuition is real.

To recap, subjects were shown randomly flash cards of pleasant or disturbing images. They reacted to the upsetting images before they appeared on the screen, their emotional reactions reflected by changes in galvanic skin response (GSR) and heart-rate variability.

The study may be less persuasive than the rich anecdotal evidence for intuition in everyday life.

British biochemist Rupert Sheldrake has been pretty well blackballed by the orthodox scientific establishment for his research on intuition, which he describes in books with intriguing titles such as *Dogs That Know When Their Owners Are Coming Home*, and *The Sense of Being Stared At*.

Sheldrake is a brilliant man. He holds a PhD in biochemistry from Cambridge, where he was a fellow of Clare College. His lectures on intuition are fascinating—several are available on YouTube.

Intuition is a hot topic, thanks to Malcolm Gladwell's bestseller, *Blink: The Power of Thinking Without Thinking*, which touts the value of following our "gut instincts."

While *Blink* is fascinating, it shares a deficiency with

Sheldrake's work: it gives us a rich catalog of intuitions that proved correct, but it doesn't suggest how we can develop our own "gut instincts."

Before we can improve our intuition, we need to understand how it works.

When are we most intuitive? When we're calm, focused, and dispassionate. Here's a meditation exercise that will help improve your intuition.

Sit in a comfortable position and close your eyes.

Inhale deeply. Tense your whole body, then quickly relax while "throwing out" the breath: "huh-huh!"

Inhale to a count of 6 to 12—whatever's comfortable. Hold the breath for the same count, and exhale to the same count again. This practice helps regularize your breathing. Calm, even breathing promotes a calm, quiet mind.

Tense and relax as in step 1, and repeat three times.

Relax and hold your attention *gently* at the point between the eyebrows. Don't strain; let your attention become quietly absorbed at that point. If you're spiritually inclined, you can offer a prayer there.

While relaxing at that point, watch your breathing, and mentally repeat a calming phrase with each inhalation and exhalation. For example, "In . . . out" or "Gather . . . relax." In yoga meditation, it's common to mentally say "hong" on inhalation and "sau" (pronounced "*saw*") on exhalation. These words are believed to have a calming effect on the nerve currents associated with inhalation and exhalation.

Don't make it a chore. Feel you're relaxing away from outward concerns, finding the center of your being, and drawing energy and inspiration from that point for your running and your life.

Feel that in going within, you're rising to greet the spirit of which you are a small expression. In that oneness, expand your heart in sympathy to all.

In meditative traditions, it's said that the more time we spend in the inner silence, the more intuitive we'll become. If you'd like to learn more about meditation, I recommend John Novak's book, *How to Meditate*, and the audio CD, *Meditation for Starters* by Kriyananda.

41. RUNNING FOR RESULTS

Alfie Kohn is the author of several interesting books on education: *No Contest: The Case Against Competition, Punished by Rewards,* and *The Schools Our Children Deserve.*

A 1987 *Boston Globe* article on Kohn's work, "Studies Find Reward Often No Motivator,"[40] cites a growing body of research that shows rewards can inhibit performance and creativity instead of improving them.

Young children who are rewarded for drawing are less likely to draw on their own than are children who draw just for the fun of it. Teenagers offered rewards for playing word games enjoy the games less and do not do as well as those who play with no rewards. Employees who are praised for meeting a manager's expectations suffer a drop in motivation.

I doubt I'm the only runner who's ever weighed the value of training for results, against the simple pleasures of running for its own sake. Confirming the research on intrinsic motivation, I find there is no conflict: I get the best results when I train to maximize enjoyment.

Kohn cites studies by Theresa Amabile, associate professor of psychology at Brandeis. Amabile found that children who were offered a reward did less creative work on art and poetry-

---

40. Alfie Kohn, "Studies Find Reward Often No Motivator," special to the *Boston Globe*, January 19, 1987.

writing projects.

I've been fortunate to meet a number of people who've been world leaders in their fields, in business, sports, science, academics, and spirituality. Without exception, they shared three qualities: they all had tremendous energy, intense, laser-like concentration, and boundless enthusiasm.

Kohn describes the joy-killing effects of chasing results. Rewards encourage people to get the job done as fast as possible, with less care, in order to get the reward.

Second, people feel less independent when working for a reward; thus their work is less creative.

Finally, people lose focus on the pleasures inherent in the work when they're focused on a reward; so they're less careful.

This is all good, ripe stuff for runners. It confirms what we know in our hearts: that when we run for results, the feeling is contractive. When we think "I'm training for the day when I'll run a 2:50 marathon," the flow of energy gets cut off and joy slips away. When we run expansively, mindful of a goal but lost in the creative joy of the moment, our energy rises.

The running magazines tell us, endlessly, how to get a reward: how to improve our 10K and marathon PRs, lose weight, and get stronger. They're filled with articles by PhDs who preach the mechanics of running—diet, intervals, injuries, shoes, heart monitors, training schedules, on and on.

But that's the external surface of the sport—it's the physical stuff we must do to achieve a future result, whether it's basic fitness or a gold medal. An equally useful science would tell us about increasing the liberating joys of "just running."

42. ART OF SPORTS, LAW OF SPORTS

Browsing at the library, I came across a wonderful set of seven DVDs, *The History of Soccer*.

I've never played soccer, and I'm not a fan, but something drew me to bring the videos home.

Aside from the spectacular game footage, the fascinating interviews with former players (oldest age 91), and the scenery of foreign lands, I was struck most powerfully by the distinction that soccer culture makes between "the Game of Art" and "the Game of Results."

It's obvious from the terms what they refer to. For years in Brazil, the tone of play was set by stars like Pelé, who played the Game of Art with incredible skill and success. It's said that the Brazilian "beautiful game" derives, in part, from *capoeira*, the native martial art which incorporates elements of dance.

Less known is that, earlier in the 20th century, the international teams from Uruguay and Argentina established even better records than Brazil eventually would, and that both countries thrived on the Game of Art. Moreover, one of the first African teams to do well in the World Cup, Cameroon, would showcase the beautiful game.

It's striking what happened when three of those countries—Argentina, Brazil, and Cameroon—switched to the Game of Results.

As Brazil became successful, European professional teams

began to lure the best Brazilian players away with offers of fat contracts. Desperate to keep succeeding, the Brazilians resorted to violent tactics intended to disrupt the competition and allow them to win at any cost. They failed miserably. Brazil descended to a second-rate power, not because its pool of talent was depleted, but because negativity kills energy, and never cancels a positive.

The same thing happened earlier in Argentina. Argentina has a large Italian population, and many of the country's stars were of Italian descent. As soon as the national team began to fare well, the Italian professional teams started hiring the stars away. Like Brazil, Argentina panicked and resorted to the Game of Results. The fans lost interest, the players grew disillusioned, the sponsors were turned off, and the media expressed disgust. Soon, Argentina was no longer a world power.

Running a 5K or a marathon competitively, as opposed to jogging it as a social fun-run, requires a seriousness of purpose and a focus on results. But it's funny how often people who are well-rounded in other dimensions of their lives, and not just athletically, tend to do well in sports.

The Heartmath studies showed that the heart can work harder with less strain when we cultivate positive feelings. So it may not hinder the superstars if they happen to be good people.

Years ago, I read a fine book, *Stealing Jesus: How Fundamentalism Betrays Christianity*. Author Bruce Bawer points out how the fundamentalists love to quote Bible passages that portray God as angry and spiteful, while they ignore Christ's central message of compassion, forgiveness, and love. Bawer distinguishes between the "Church of Law" and the "Church of Love."

These "churches" are reflected in our own nature. Looking back, I can see times in my life when I've joined the Church of Law. And I recognize that every time I've done something I cringe to remember, it was because I lacked love. Conversely, everything I've done that I'm proud of, I did as a member of the Church of Love.

Human history is the story of the struggle between these two opposing urges in us. Every good book, movie, or play is about these issues.

In my running, I find that I make the best progress, and have the best experiences, when I run with a heart attuned to universal currents of love. My worst runs are those where I leave the Church of Love—where I'm too hard on myself, or I abuse my body by going too fast or far. Fortunately, those mistakes are increasingly rare, because I know that a positive trumps a negative every time. When I play the Game of Art, I have more fun, and the results come more easily.

43. THE RUNNER'S BRAIN

A tire on my car developed a bubble—*thump, thump*—and I went to Wheel Works for a replacement. They said it would take an hour, so I strolled to Target to look at sweatshirts, then returned to the waiting room and thumbed through a copy of *U.S. News*. The back cover featured an Allstate ad with an illustration of a brain. The caption asked rhetorically if 16-year-olds are missing part of their brain.

I'm fascinated by a field of research that's been popularly dubbed "neurotheology." It includes studies of what happens in the brains of people who meditate, and in states that subjects describe as "spiritual experiences."

As I've noted in previous chapters, an area of the brain that becomes activated in meditators is the prefrontal cortex (PFC), just behind the forehead. It's the "young" part of the brain, where uniquely human attributes are localized. That part of the brain doesn't develop fully until our early twenties. It's a serious problem for young drivers: 16-year-olds have three times as many crashes as 17-year-olds, five times as many as 18-year-olds.

Allstate wants state governments to create Graduated Driver Licensing (GDL) laws to reduce teen crashes. The laws would restrict teens from nighttime driving and driving with other teen passengers. When North Carolina implemented strict GDL laws, crash rates for 16-year-olds dropped 25%.

Not long ago, a friend and I reminisced over lunch about the idiotic way we drove almost 60 years ago, when a key part of our brains was missing.

Bruce remembered racing through suburban Phoenix streets at over 100 mph. I remembered flying (yes, we were airborne) over Arizona desert back roads in the 1954 Cadillac of a local doctor, his mentally defective 16-year-old son at the wheel, and in a 1928 Ford Model A that belonged to another of my pals. I remembered zooming up an incredibly steep hill in Bruce's WWII-era Jeep, whereupon the Jeep flipped and we spilled out, fortunate that it didn't land on top of us.

Perhaps teenagers should be taught to meditate. It might save lives. Various meditative traditions teach that by concentrating attention gently in the prefrontal cortex, we can develop the abilities that neuroscientists associate with that area, including emotional maturity and calm concentration.

Richard J. Davidson, PhD, is a leading expert on the prefrontal cortex. Davidson is Professor of Psychology and Psychiatry and Director of the University of Wisconsin's Laboratory of Affective Neuroscience.

In *Visions of Compassion: Western Scientists and Tibetan Buddhists Examine Human Nature*, Davidson reports:

Of particular note in this regard are pilot data collected . . . in one older monk who had been engaged in daily practices to cultivate compassion for more than 30 years. We measured brain electrical activity during the baseline state in this monk and found that he exhibited the most extreme left prefrontal activation compared with a normative sample of 175 Wisconsin students.

Scientists tend to be cautious in their statements. In plain language, what Davidson is saying is that, in competition with 175 college students, the meditating monk's left prefrontal cortex scored off the chart. And because left-prefrontal activation is associated with positive affective states, his test score indicated that he was a happy dude.

How can this research help runners? One "ability" of the PFC that's particularly useful, as I mentioned earlier, is emotional control.

I described how brain scientists have found that raw, uncontrolled emotions are localized in an older structure of the brain, the amygdala. There are strong neural connections between the forebrain and amygdala, and the scientists have found that energizing one structure *withdraws* energy from the other. Thus when we concentrate deeply, the PFC becomes activated and pulls energy away from raw emotions in the amygdala. It's the physiological basis for the age-old maxim that when we're under emotional stress, we need to focus—"keep busy."

I think it's wonderful that Allstate suggests we regulate teenage zombies. The facts don't lie: 18-year-olds have one-fifth as many wrecks as 16-year-olds.

Surely, sports training in the future will draw on these and other brain findings.

These ideas have been a feature of spiritual teachings for millennia. In Western religious art, saints are shown gazing upward, toward the "spiritual eye." In the East, artists paint the saints with a mark at the center of the forehead, above and between the eyebrows. The practice of energizing the prefrontal cortex is referred to in the scriptures.

From the Bible:

> "If thine eye be single, thy body shall be full of light."
> (Matthew 6:22)

And the Bhagavad Gita (from *The Song Celestial: Bhagavad-Gita*, translated by Sir Edwin Arnold):

> His gaze absorbed
> Upon his nose–end [the origin of the nose, at the point
> between the eyebrows], rapt from all around,
> Tranquil in spirit, free of fear, intent
> Upon his Brahmacharya vow, devout,
> Musing on Me, lost in the thought of Me.
> That Yogin, so devoted, so controlled,
> Comes to the peace beyond—My peace, the peace
> Of high Nirvana!

44. HOW PREFONTAINE TRAINED

Kenny Moore was a teammate of Steve Prefontaine's at the University of Oregon. In the marathon at the 1972 Olympics where Frank Shorter won gold, Moore finished fourth.

Moore's book, *Bowerman and the Men of Oregon: The Story of Oregon's Legendary Coach and Nike's Cofounder*, gives us a wonderful insider's look at how Oregon became a collegiate powerhouse. It's packed with revealing stories and insights.

Am I the only runner who's ever wondered if the training methods of highly elite athletes are relevant for me?

In an interview with *Runner's World Daily News*, sports physiologist David L. Costill observed that world-class runners and ordinary Joes like us are so different as to be almost unique species. The physiological differences are huge.

I experienced this firsthand on a spring day on the campus of Stanford University. Stanford is a wonderful place to run—it has 3000 acres of tree-lined streets and grassy, oak-dotted hills.

I was running 2-minute repeats as hard as I could in my sad old-man's body, probably at 6:30 pace, when I heard the pitter-patter of runners approaching from behind.

It was a herd of Stanford's NCAA-champion distance runners. The group included 2000 Olympian Brad Hauser, twin brother Brent, and 5000-meter NCAA champion Ian Dobson.

They passed me effortlessly—they weren't even breathing hard. At six-minute pace, they were warming up for a track race.

Okay, I was in my early sixties and ran like an aardvark. But it was humbling.

While reading Kenny Moore's book, I was struck by how relevant Bowerman's methods are for all runners, including my ancient self. Bowerman was successful because he discovered core principles that anyone can apply.

Moore reports that Bowerman never got lost in the details. He didn't prescribe rigid, numbers-based workouts. Instead, he studied what each athlete could do and assigned workouts accordingly. Prefontaine's amazing body allowed him to train hard several days in a row, while Moore needed a hard/easy schedule, with one brutally hard run every two weeks.

Here's how Moore describes Bowerman's training. Does it apply to you?

Bowerman began exhorting Oregon runners to finish their workouts "exhilarated, not exhausted." As he timed them on interval days, he would scrutinize their form, grabbing a runner's throat and taking his pulse. He'd check the glint in their eye, sending the tight and dull to the showers, and especially those whose pulses weren't quick to return to 120 beats per minute. His credo was that it was better to underdo than overdo. He was adamant that he trained individuals, not teams, and he came to believe that group workouts could even be counterproductive. "The best man loafs, the worst tears himself down," he would say. "Maybe only one guy in the middle gets the optimum work."

This was the foundation of his annual welcoming address to incoming freshmen.

"Stress, recover, improve, that's all training is," he'd say. "You'd think any damn fool could do it." In fact, interval training takes such care that to this day few coaches can consistently produce milers.

Elsewhere, I've celebrated Bill Walsh, the coach who led the San Francisco 49ers to three Super Bowl victories in the 1980s.

Walsh had a lot in common with Bowerman. Both built their success on understanding the individual. Walsh never treated his players as spare parts, to be bought and discarded according to how well they could be welded into the team machine. He got the best out of each player, because he took the trouble to understand them. Kenny Moore makes it clear that Bowerman took the same approach.

The title of this chapter is misleading. I haven't told you how Pre trained—how many miles, how many intervals, what pace, etc. I'm fine with that, because I don't see how it could possibly help you.

Many runners who read the great Arthur Lydiard's books complain, "He doesn't give us the details." To repeat—how much good would it do us, if he did? Optimal training is never a question of deciding to run a fixed effort and sticking to the plan regardless. That's foolhardy. The best training is where you listen to your unique body and adjust the pace and duration accordingly, moment by moment. And if your body tells you to pack it in and go home, good training happens when you're sufficiently honest and disciplined and mentally tough to comply.

I used to think that "feeling-based training," as advocated by Bowerman and Lydiard, and practiced by champions like Frank Shorter, was a copout. "Run how you feel" evoked wishy-washy images of quitters and slobs. In a whiny voice:

"I train how I feel, and if I don't feel like it, I won't run."

Listening to the body is demanding. It's *not* easy to obey the body's signals—to run slowly when the body craves rest and impatient emotions want to do more. Bowerman, Lydiard, and Walsh trained hundreds of successful athletes, and not one of them said it was easy.

These great coaches gave us important answers: You've got to be tough, and you've got to listen.

45. HAPPY HEART RUNNING

It isn't every day a runner is blessed to cruise effortlessly for mile after mile, at a lickety-split pace while bathing in inner peace and joy. And it's especially rare if he's in his sixties. Yet in the last month it's been my good fortune to run in that blissful state not once but three times. Here's what happened on the first run.

I set out from the Stanford football stadium and jogged my usual warmup through the sports complex, past the swimming pools, baseball and soccer fields, and through a lovely eucalyptus grove.

I started the run with a firm affirmation. "I don't want to run for any other reason than to expand my heart. I don't want to run for personal glory, or to run fast so that others will admire me. That would be stealing from them. I want to run to discover my heart and radiate kindness and goodwill to all."

I warmed up for an entire hour. Wary of falling into the trap of running too fast, I held my heart rate at 65–70% of maximum. That's quite slow, a shuffle, but I was determined not to run faster until my heart told me my body was ready.

For the first 40 minutes, I struggled with restless thoughts. As I sought a mental focus, my heart and mind began to relax and feel at peace. Jogging through the biology complex and finding my rhythm, a Duke Ellington lyric popped into my mind: *"It don't mean a thing if it ain't got that swing!"*

As my pace slowly climbed, I glanced at the heart monitor. I was running at a speed that would normally raise my heart to 77–78% of max, yet it was cruising at 70–72%. What happened? Obviously, it meant I was fit and rested. I wondered if the long warmup had also given my body time to become nicely synchronized.

An hour into the run, my body felt as if it could happily run faster, and I let it accelerate. All the while, I checked to be sure I was making the right decisions. I knew I could easily slip into running too fast, and I steadfastly curbed the impulse.

With the stopwatch at 1:02, I asked my intuition if I should run fast or go long. Sensing no clear answer, I decided to try some fast running and see how it felt.

I picked up the pace, and as my pulse rose I checked the feeling in my heart. As my heart rate passed 80% of maximum, I noticed a distinct feeling of harmony; but as it climbed to 85% and beyond, the feeling faded. I held pace at 85–87% for a few minutes. Then I thought, "If I don't drop back to 80% and explore those good feelings, I might miss an opportunity to learn something wonderful."

I slowed until my heart fell to 80%, and for three miles I held that pace and was rewarded with extraordinary feelings of harmony and joy.

At the start of the run, I'd had trouble finding a rhythm as I struggled to pull my thoughts together and lift my mood. Now, a lovely rhythm came effortlessly. My body was poised over its center, my feet padding lightly over the ground. My spine was straight and my breathing was deep and expansive, filling my upper body. My head was raised calmly, eyes relaxed and looking straight ahead. My attention was strongly interiorized—I had no trouble keeping my mind focused while running on the verge of a busy road with cars whizzing by. It was pleasant to remain "inside," while the world "out there" went its way—it simply didn't matter. This was a delightful way to run. The thought came irresistibly: *"This is Happy Heart running."*

Today I *knew* how to train. It felt so completely *right*, and the knowing came from my heart, with undeniable certainty. I ran expansively, and the proof was that my heart was more than physically and emotionally soothed. There were feelings of a love and joy that, after the run, I found I could extend to others. On the way home I stopped at the market, and as I chatted with the checkout clerk my heart was relaxed and appreciative, glowing with unspoken kindness.

An hour and a half into the run, I swung back through the campus, in a long S-curve past the Quad and through the biology complex. My body had begun to tire, and it announced the fact by running slower at the same heart rate. But that was fine; I felt no compulsion to force my body to run faster. The heart's love was all-sufficing; I didn't need to prove anything.

Today I knew how to train. I knew when to start running faster, and I knew exactly how fast to run. There was the first, fleeting harmony in my heart when it passed 80%, as if to say *"That's it!"* And the confirmation, with miles of running in primal happiness, my heart bathed in joy. Afterward, there was the proof—my body worked hard, doing *good* training, and my spirit sang through the deep channels of my body.

It was, in every respect, a perfect run. It was excellent training, it was mentally healing, and it was spiritually blessed.

46. THE 96% RUN

I rose early and drove to San Francisco. On the freeway I sang happily, and when I parked at Crissy Field next to the Bay I was in fine spirits.

I set off at a slow trot toward the Golden Gate Bridge, working to focus my mind, relax my heart, and attune myself to the right kind of running for the day.

It was a gorgeous mid-November morning in the City—sunny and warm at 9 AM, not a cloud in the sky. Climbing the gentle slope of the bridge, I kept my heart rate at around 68% of maximum. Halfway across, I felt warmed up and let it rise to 75%.

When my attention wandered, I brought it gently back to a focus, while I relaxed and practiced spiritual mindfulness at the point between the eyebrows. As I've mentioned, various spiritual traditions tell us that the "spiritual eye" is the physical center of concentration, and the "broadcast station" for sending prayers. Paintings of saints show them with uplifted eyes. Neuroscientists know that the prefrontal cortex is where the most advanced human abilities are localized in the brain, such as will power, concentration, perseverance, and the ability to achieve goals and hold positive attitudes. They've discovered that the anterior cingulate gyrus, a brain structure within the center of the forehead, becomes activated in meditative states.

The world's scriptures mention many connections between bodily centers and spiritual states. The Catholic saint, Teresa of Avila, said that she experienced ecstasy at the top of the brain—the "crown chakra" of Eastern lore.

Trotting down the north slope of the bridge, I reminded myself to "relax in the heart," and as I did so I felt my heart softly open, as if a gate had swung wide. Certain spiritual teachings speak of the heart as the "receiving station" where we receive God's answers to our prayers. Many spiritual practices aim at opening the heart, such as the "prayer of the heart" of Eastern Orthodoxy, the devotional chanting of the East, and the dancing of Native Americans and Sufis.

Coming off the bridge, my heart was cruising comfortably at 77%. I stopped briefly in the restroom and saw a young runner tending to bloody knees. He said he'd fallen on the Coastal Trail, but it wasn't as bad as it looked. I said it looked pretty bad and wished him a good run.

I descended to the pedestrian crosswalk under the bridge, then jogged onto the Coastal Trail. The running felt easy as I ascended the switchbacks to the crest of the Marin Headlands. I walked the final, very steep section, then descended by the paved road that winds back down to the bridge, enjoying the amazing views of the ocean, Golden Gate, and City.

Back on the bridge, I thought about doing some tempo running, but decided it would be foolish—the run would be over two hours, and I'd promised a friend that I would be ready to go hiking in the afternoon. I relaxed in my heart and resolved to let the "inside" decide how I should run.

Shortly before the first bridge tower, about a quarter of the way across, I found myself running at tempo pace effortlessly, while feeling inwardly focused and harmonious. My heart rate was about 88–90% of maximum, yet it felt sweet and easeful. It was very unusual, because while running at such a high heart rate, I'm normally aware of the effort—it feels "uncomfortably hard."

I'd enjoyed that state of effortless ease for a while when I glanced at the heart monitor and saw that I was running at 92% of MHR. Wow, that was flying! I backed off momentarily, but a quiet intuition urged me to run even faster.

Praying that I wasn't deceiving myself into running like a maniac, I brought the pace back to 92%, and soon I was cruising at 94%, then 96% of MHR, and it was completely easy—I wasn't breathing hard at all, and there was no sensation of pain. My mind wasn't struggling or tense; in fact, it was completely calm. I was in a state of silence, where thinking seemed superfluous, a distraction. It was deeply enjoyable, although it didn't have the same quality of heart-joy that I had experienced, at a lower heart rate, during the "Happy Heart Run" described in the last chapter. I decided this wasn't Happy Heart running, but something else.

As I continued to run at 96% of MHR, I recalled that, while running across the bridge the previous weekend, I'd talked inwardly to my spiritual teacher and asked how it's possible to run aerobically at a very high heart rate, as the top marathoners do. Did that ability come only after years of running hundred-mile weeks? Was that the sacrifice required to fulfill the runner's dream of effortlessly flight?

In *Running: The Athlete Within*, pioneering sports physiologist David Costill reports that some Olympic-class marathoners are able to run *aerobically* at 90% of their maximum heart rate (MHR) and even higher. It's a figure that boggles the brain, because most physiologists consider an average, non-elite runner's "aerobic training pace" to be 60% to 75% of max.

For most runners, 90% feels uncomfortably labored and can't be sustained for long. Yet here I was, at age 60, running at 96% of MHR with a calm mind and relaxed and steady heart. (Of course, the great ones can do it for 26.2 miles, at 4:55 pace!)

Yet, granting my pedestrian gifts, how was it possible? I'm convinced that it had physical, mental, emotional, and spiritual dimensions. I'm certain, for example, that it was possible, in part, because I took a long warmup and used the time to focus my mind, open my heart, ask for inner guidance, and follow the guidance that came.

I suspect that a key factor was fine-tuning my heart. In their research on heart-brain-body "coherence," the scientists at HeartMath Institute discovered that zone-like states can occur at any heart rate—what counts isn't the *speed* of the heartbeat, but the *pattern*. Disharmonious feelings such as anger and hatred make the heart beat with an inefficient, erratic rhythm at any speed ("incoherently," as the researchers put it). When we're angry, upset, depressed, etc., the heart changes speed chaotically. But positive feelings make the heart change speeds "coherently" and harmoniously—the heart beats at a steady, harmonious, rhythmically changing rate. Graphs of heart-rate variability reveal these coherent and incoherent patterns—the curves generated in negative states are visibly jangly and disharmonious, while the images generated in states of love, kindness, etc., are smooth and regular. (See figure 1, chapter 5.)

I'm convinced there was also a physical foundation for what I experienced. For months, I had done nearly all my runs at an easy, aerobic pace, and then I had introduced a weekly twenty-minute tempo run at 85–92% MHR.

Later, when I mentioned this experience on an Internet

forum, several people questioned if I had measured my maximum heart rate accurately.

In fact, I'd followed the standard protocol to the letter, warming up with several miles of easy running, followed by a mile on the track at a hard pace, then two nearly all-out half-miles, and finally, a full-out quarter-mile. My heart rate measured 174 on the monitor, and I couldn't make it budge, even by running up the stadium stairs as hard as I could.

Coming off the bridge, I slowed in the parking lot, which was clogged with tourists, then picked up the pace on the road down to the bayside. Normally, at this point I would slow to a jog, but there was no suggestion of fatigue, and I continued to run effortlessly at 96% MHR.

Toward the end of the run, I decided to try an experiment: I would run all-out, as hard as I could, and see what it felt like. Would I experience the raw pain of the maximum heart rate test run? Or would my heart retain some vestige of relaxed, harmonious feeling? I broke into a full sprint, and my heart swiftly rose to 175 and wouldn't go higher. There was a feeling of struggle, but it was nothing like the pain I'd endured during the all-out test run. The feeling in my heart wasn't notably harmonious, but it wasn't disharmonious, either.

The sequel is that I recovered very quickly. On the day after such a taxing effort, I would normally feel nervy and on edge, and on the second day I would feel sleepy in the afternoon, incapable of mental work. But this time there was no letdown. I drank tons of water for the remainder of the day, and it may have helped my recovery, but after other hard runs, not even drinking like a fish had prevented the "second-day blahs."

I came across an article recently about Eddy Merckx, the

legendary Belgian who won the Tour de France five times in the 1960s and '70s. The article described how Merckx would warm up with no less than 20 to 30 miles of easy riding before each Tour stage. The other riders, meanwhile, were only too happy to catch a ride to the start, intent on conserving their energy. It's easy to imagine them shaking their heads as Merckx pedaled by. Yet I wonder if the long warmups didn't contribute to Eddy's success. They were, in fact, about an hour and twenty minutes, roughly the duration of my warmup during the 96% run.

On the weekends that followed, I returned to San Francisco, hoping to repeat the experience and learn more about the art of fast, effortless running. But those runs were qualified successes, at best.

I repeated the steps in the same order—focusing attention, working to open my heart, etc. And I was able to run at 96% of MHR effortlessly—but with little enjoyment.

Those runs were disappointing. I was grasping at the experience, instead of cultivating it with a sincere heart, immersed in the moment, accepting whatever would come. I *wanted* it too much—and my wanting was tainted by a galloping selfishness. With one part of my mind I *did* want to let go of ego and run selflessly in the "now," but with another I was focused on results, living in the future, unable to immerse myself in the present.

On the first 96% run, I did a good job of preparing the five tools of a runner to perform at a high level. My body was well-trained and rested, and during the long warmup I focused on harmonizing my heart, concentrating my willpower and attention, and offering myself humbly to receive the soul's guidance. I wasn't expecting anything. I was completely content to enjoy the moment, free of craving.

Not an easy state to achieve!

What's it worth to run fast without genuine enjoyment, if all I accomplish is to run with cold physical speed? Those runs taught me a valuable lesson. No amount of physical success can satisfy me. The best rewards of "spiritual running" have come when I've succeeded in purifying my heart.

47. NIGHTINGALE

Three times in the last 18 months, I've had an easy run. Woo-woo! Isn't that special?!

It typically goes like this. It's a lovely Saturday morning, and I drive into the hills feeling wonderful. But, once out on the trail, my energy goes blooey.

It's happened with stupefying regularity for a year and a half. And it's always the same: I begin the run feeling awful, but in the back of my mind there's an inner voice that says, *"If you persevere with indomitable will, you'll be able to rise above this experience, and you'll come out of it feeling fine."* Every run has been a struggle, but many have ended well.

I drove 50 miles north to the beautiful coastal mountains of Marin County, feeling ghastly. I was dizzy with malaise. When I stopped at Tam Junction to buy bottled water, I was so weary that my neck ached. But I sensed a still, small voice that told me to go to Muir Woods and begin the run regardless.

The climb from Muir Woods to the ridge above Pantoll is beautiful—three miles on a dirt road that ascends an unrelenting 2000 feet through redwood forests and lovely meadows, with intermittent views over the ocean. But today it was a terrible slog. Belabored by physical unease, mind babbling, feeling fretful and ill, I looked forward to turning around at the ranger station and trundling back to the truck in limp-home mode. But when I reached Pantoll, the interior voice told me to keep going.

I jogged up the paved highway toward the ridge tops. As I slowly ascended on the margin of the road, I heard the sound of bagpipes coming apparently from the foggy woods below. As I rounded a bend, I saw a group of people gathered on a grassy knoll. They were dressed in formal attire: dark suits for the men, white dresses for the women. They were too far away to tell what they were doing, but the bagpipes suggested a memorial service. Were they mourning a departed friend? A beloved pet? At the trailhead, a card tacked to a fencepost gave directions to the Miller wedding.

I swung onto the steepest trail that led upward to the ridgetop. After climbing a hundred feet, I turned and looked down on the wedding party, which was set in a stunning scene. The bagpipes played "Wild Mountain Thyme." The little party stood in a circle, the bride in her white dress, as wisps of fog played tag with the sun, with wonderful views south to San Francisco and the Bay, and north over rolling hills to Point Reyes. I let my heart bathe in the beauty of the scene and sent silent prayers of blessing to the newlyweds.

Reaching the ridge, I traversed the lovely single-track trails that crisscross the steep meadows, before turning back down toward Pantoll. I felt somewhat better mentally, but my body was still explicitly tired.

Arriving at Pantoll, I felt no enthusiasm for returning by the route I had ascended, and I wondered if there was another downward trail that I could explore. I was reconciling myself to taking the fire road, when I noticed a trailhead from the parking lot. A sign said Steep Ravine Trail. I recalled that a friend had said it was a special place.

I've never seen a more lovely mountain ravine—it

reminded me of the jungle trails of Kauai, but it was more beautiful for being crisp and cool rather than languorously tropical. The trail descended at a moderate slope for three miles, shaded throughout, hugging a cheerful stream that ran full. Mossy trees, huge ferns, and a plant with tall green stems and huge, platter-like leaves made a mythic scene.

Amid the beauty, my mood was reserved. I was deeply enjoying this wonderful place, but in a way that was inward and quiet. I had won a tough battle over my miserable, faltering body, and I felt not much inclined to reinvest in its questionable joys. It was enough to *feel* this illusory glory, and enjoy it from within.

I was aware that if I couldn't find a trail over the hill to Muir Woods, I would have to climb the dreaded stairs of the Dipsea Trail. I met a pair of hikers and asked about a cross-trail, but they only babbled incoherently. I decided to enjoy Steep Ravine and face the Dipsea when I got there. The inner voice whispered that I'd be okay if I remained rooted in this stillness.

Turning onto the Dipsea, I crossed the footbridge to the base of the stairs and began waddling up them at a fair pace, using an energy-saving sideways roll I'd discovered during the Quadruple Dipsea race.

I was amazed by how much it helped, physically and mentally, to stay calm and inward. I had enjoyed the descent of Steep Ravine in that quiet state, and while sweating up the stairs I continued to rest in that silent cave. I thought, "Perhaps this is where the months of lousy runs were leading; perhaps I'm learning to subdue the body and win inner joy."

I had long since discovered that God didn't care about making my runs easy. Always there had been problems. Every good run had come at a price—there had been no free passes, and very few days when running was effortless. The exceptions were notable. On the morning of the lottery for the 1997 Western States Hundred-Mile Endurance Run, I ran light as a feather, sailing effortlessly up a long hill, knowing with calm certainty that my name had been drawn. When a friend phoned with the news, hours later, I interrupted him: "I know."

Logic told me that running ought to get easier with time, as experience and training merge to make each run more blissful than the last. And God had simply laughed. He tested me in His kindness, because there is no joy without continual expansion.

I understood that the lesson of running isn't about creating good runs, but learning to be happy even when running turns brutal. I haven't mastered the art of unconquerable joy, but I've become somewhat more attuned to the process, and my successes come more often.

I've bitched and raged at my bad runs. I've analyzed them, wondering if my attitude was wrong, or my diet was to blame. I've prayed impatiently, and I've scratched with the rational mind for answers. I've blamed myself for the bad runs, and I've been ashamed of them. But God isn't big on explanations. He prefers to teach us through our experiences, guiding us to ice cream, if that's what we need, or through brambles if it's the shortest path to clarity and joy.

Often I've been tempted to dismiss these months as wasted time. But now I'm grateful. God is a surgeon who doesn't shrink from inflicting pain to save the patient.

I'm grateful. I no longer shy from hard runs, as I might have two years ago. My hard experiences now hold a promise of great joy.

Composer Donald Walters said it beautifully in his "Song

of the Nightingale":

> *Nightingale, nightingale*
> *Sing of joy through the night.*
> *Teach all men how to spin*
>   *Clouds of gloom into light.*
> *Without silence, what is song?*
> *Without night, where is dawn?*
> *Were it not for men's woes,*
> *Who would smile at a rose?*

Newcomers to running are enticed by enjoyment of one kind, while experienced runners seek more sophisticated pleasures. What begins as a fitness quest, ends as a quest for joy. The inner athlete becomes the enduringly real athlete. Whether the body is injured or running strongly, our attention drifts over the years to running's inner lessons, lessons that bring deeper joys than our fleeting outward successes can yield. The runner gradually ascends from the body, through the heart, to the soul.

RESOURCES

To share your thoughts, please email me: gbeinhorn@ gmail.com. I'd love to hear from you. Or you can use the contact form at www.joyfulathlete.com.

Body

Here's my choice for the best book on training for distance runners: *Healthy Intelligent Training: The Proven Principles of Arthur Lydiard*, by Keith Livingstone. It's the Lydiard Foundation's recommended textbook, and it's completely faithful to Lydiard's philosophy and methods. Best of all, it includes many stories that convey the spirit of the New Zealand running scene where Lydiard's ideas were first proved.

Lore of Running. Tim Noakes, MD. The single best source on the science and practice of running. This 900-page book includes many engaging stories of great runners and their training, plus reliable information on injuries, diet, etc.

Diet Books. I've never found a diet book that got it completely right. The problem is, they're biased. An author discovers that low carbs, low fat, or an exotic herb can help people lose fat, and then it becomes an intolerant religion.

Eating for high energy requires balance. It's a no-brainer: the body doesn't thrive on one-sided diets that overemphasize carbs, fats, or anything else.

That much said, *Eat to Live*, by Joel Fuhrman, MD, will tell you, in crystal-clear detail, exactly why fruits and veggies are good for you. It's the best weight-loss book I've found. The Eat to Live diet is healthy, easy, tasty, and sustainable, and it's based on hard research from reputable sources. I do have quibbles with the diet. I'm suspicious of one-sided arguments against saturated fats, dairy products, and seafood. Otherwise, it's an outstanding guide to rapid, easy, healthy weight-loss.

The Ayurvedic Cookbook, and *Ayurvedic Cooking for Westerners*. Amadea Morningstar and Urmila Desai. Ayurveda is an ancient dietary system from India. It's valuable for athletes, because it identifies foods that can create problems for people of a particular body "type," and foods that will help us feel physically, emotionally, and mentally balanced.

Heart

I'm indebted to Joe Henderson, the editor who nurtured *Runner's World* through its best years. I felt very alone as a runner until I found Joe's writing, in 1972. A "writer's writer," widely admired for his enjoyable, clean style, Joe's articles and books spoke in the authentic voice of runners everywhere. I rejoice that two of his classics are now available on Amazon (at bargain prices!).

Long Slow Distance: The Human Way to Train (originally published in 1969). This book created a sports acronym that all runners now recognize: *LSD*. The late George Sheehan said: "Joe Henderson is a revolutionary not because his writings have produced a wave of faster runners, but because he has spawned happier ones." It's a great read, not just for the liberating method, but for the wonderful stories of old-time revolutionaries: Boston winner Amby Burfoot, U.S. 50-

mile champion Bob Deines, ultrarunning legend Tom Osler, and others.

Long Run Solution: What I Like Best About Running and Do Most as a Runner (originally published in 1976). Nobody said it better about *Long Run Solution* than Rich Benyo, the editor of *Marathon & Beyond*: "There isn't a five-year period in which I don't pick up *Long Run Solution* and read it again, both to bring back the energizing effect of validating long-distance running as an adult pursuit and as an antidote to a too-pressured, too-stressed life."

My Personal Best: Life Lessons from an All-American Journey. John Wooden. Possibly the most inspiring sports book ever written, in a close race with Phil Jackson's *Eleven Rings*. Wooden describes the early life experiences that led him to create his "Pyramid of Success," a chart of values that guided and inspired the 10 NCAA-champion basketball teams he coached at UCLA.

Eleven Rings: The Soul of Success. Phil Jackson. Jackson's memoir of his life as a basketball player and coach at the highest level doesn't have a single boring page. There aren't many nonfiction books that I've been able to read happily in long stretches, but this is one. Not only highly entertaining, it's deeply revealing. How was Jackson able to meld superstars Michael Jordan, Scottie Pippen, Dennis Rodman, Kobe Bryant, and Shaquille O'Neal into bands of warrior-brothers, instead of preening prima donnas? In his relaxed, natural style, Jackson reveals how it was done. This inspiring book shows us why expansive values are the best foundation for success in any field, not just basketball.

Values of the Game. Bill Bradley. The former US senator and Hall of Fame NBA player (he played on two championship teams with the New York Knicks) shares his thoughts on courage, discipline, resilience, respect, and the joy of the game. This is a sports book for the ages.

Shooting from the Outside, by Tara VanDerveer. A wonderful account of Tara's year as coach of the 1996 U.S. women's Olympic basketball team that won 60 games without a loss on its way to the gold medal.

The Runner and the Path. Dean Ottati. Heartfelt stories from the life of an unusually aware runner. A former world-class swimmer, Dean is a successful business executive. On the trail with running friends, he finds meaning to balance the absurdities of modern corporate life.

Will

Training with the Legends. Michael Sandrock. A perceptive book that reveals the lives and training of world-class runners. Sandrock conveys the effort required to rise to the top—the talent, sacrifice, and years of hard work.

Mind

Focused for Soccer. Bill Beswick. Wonderful insights into the mental aspects of sports, from a psychologist for top English professional teams, including Manchester United.

Mental Training for Peak Performance. Steven Ungerleider, PhD. An excellent introduction to sports psychology, based on research and interviews with top athletes.

Soul

For the "deep ideas" in *Joyful Athlete,* I'm deeply grateful to J. Donald Walters for the following books. All are available from Crystal Clarity Publishers (www.crystalclarity.com).

Out of the Labyrinth: For Those Who Want to Believe, But Can't. Walters takes on the leading sourpusses of Western thought, including Jean Paul Sartre and his followers who've misinterpreted the findings of modern science and their implications. Walters demonstrates that the same findings reflect life's deep meaningfulness. An engaging, readable book for college-educated readers.

Hope for a Better World! The Small Communities Solution. A clear overview of Western thought, its promise and wrong directions taken—and an inspiring, practical prescription for a meaningful way of life.

Education for Life. Not just for parents and teachers, this book will speak to anyone who's seeking life's meaning. It describes the six-year stages of a child's development, and how to help children learn the required lessons. Adults will find inspiration for filling gaps in their own upbringing.

Intuition for Starters. A first-rate book on intuition from the practical perspective of yoga. Includes tips for developing our intuition, and for knowing the difference between intuitive guidance and false subconscious "inspiration."

Meditation for Starters. The best concise guide to meditation I've found. Offers a clear overview of techniques for calming and focusing the mind, letting go of emotional tension and worries, and deepening spiritual awareness.

ABOUT THE AUTHOR

George Beinhorn started running in 1968. Four years later, he took a job at *Runner's World*, where he served as an assistant editor and staff photographer for four years. He has raced at distances from 100 yards to 100K (62.2 miles). At age 73, he continues to explore the joys of expansive sports as a participant and observer.